# BACK TO
# *House of Health*

### REJUVENATING RECIPES TO
## *Alkalize and Energize for Life!*

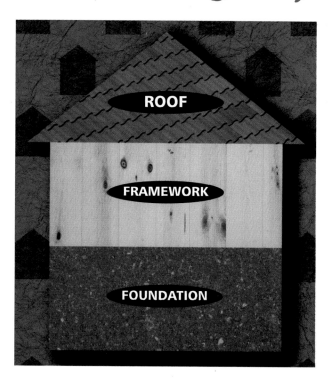

## Shelley Redford Young, L.M.T.

### with Robert O. Young, Ph.D., D.Sc.

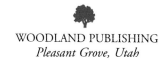

WOODLAND PUBLISHING
*Pleasant Grove, Utah*

# BACK TO THE
# *House of Health*

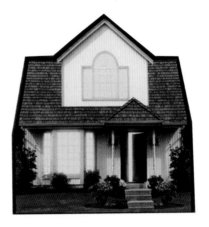

Published by Woodland Publishing
P.O. Box 160
Pleasant Grove, Utah 84062
(800) 777-2665
www.woodlandbooks.com

Editor: Dhyani Jo Sinclair
Photography by Stefan Hallberg

Printed in the United States of America.

Note: The information in this book is for educational purposes only and is not recommended as a means of diagnosing or treating an illness. All matters concerning physical and mental health should be supervised by a health practitioner knowledgeable in treating that particular condition. Neither the publisher nor author directly or indirectly dispense medical advice, nor do they prescribe any remedies or assume any responsibility for those who choose to treat themselves.

# Contents

## Recipe Titles by Alphabetical Order

## Recipe Titles by Alphabetical Order (cont.)

# Recipe Titles by Nutritional Category

# *Foreword*

The universe seems to operate by keeping opposites in balance. This I call the "Law of Opposites." For example, hot vs. cold, war vs. peace, competition vs. cooperation, disorganization vs. organization, imbalance vs. balance, darkness vs. light—and in all organized matter, acid vs. alkaline. When things get out of balance, a sign usually appears to make it known, like a headache or stomachache. One of the best examples of this principle at work is health. Health is balance in an organized system of organized, alkalized matter.

Think of your body as a fish tank. Think of the importance of maintaining the integrity of the internal fluids of the body that we "swim" in daily. Imagine the fish in this tank are your cells and organ systems bathed in fluids, which transport food and remove wastes.

Now, imagine I back up a car and put the tailpipe up against the air intake filter that supplies the oxygen for the water in the tank. The water becomes filled with carbon monoxide, lowering the alkaline pH, creating an acidic pH environment, and threatening the health of the "fish," your cells and organs.

What if I throw in too much food or the wrong kind of food (acid-producing food like dairy, sugar, and animal protein) and the fish are unable to consume or digest it all, and it starts to decompose and putrefy? Toxic acid waste and chemicals build up as the food breaks downs, creating more acidic by-products, altering the optimum alkaline pH.

Well, basically, this is a small example of what we may be doing to our internal fluids every day. We are fouling them with pollution (smoking?), drugs, excessive intake of food, over-consumption of acid-forming foods, and any number of transgressions which compromise the delicate balance of our internal alkaline fluids.

Some of us have fish tanks (bodies) that are barely able to support life, yet we somehow manage to struggle from day to day, building more severe imbalances until there is the inevitable crash and debilitating chronic, disturbing, and disorganizing symptomatology to deal with.

The pH level of our internal fluids affects every cell in our bodies. Extended acid imbalances of any kind are not well tolerated by the body. Indeed, the entire metabolic process depends on a balanced internal alkaline environment. A chronically over-acidic pH corrodes body tissue, slowly eating into the 60,000 miles of veins and arteries like acid eating into marble. If left unchecked, it will interrupt all cellular activities and functions, from the beating of your heart to the neural firing of your brain. Over-acidification interferes with life itself, leading to all sickness and dis-ease!

Fundamentally, all regulatory mechanisms (including breathing, circulation, digestion, hormone production, etc.) serve the purpose of balancing the internal alkaline environment, removing normally metabolized acids from body tissues without damaging healthy living cells.

What causes an acid internal environment in our body fluids? Wrong diet, a high-stress lifestyle, and toxic thinking are the main influences. A healthy, plant-based diet and low-stress lifestyle will maintain a balanced, alkaline terrain. The most fundamental of all balancing rules is this:

- The right kind of food (nutrition) is the most important single factor in the promotion of internal alkaline balance or health; and
- The wrong kind of food is the single most important factor in the promotion of biological acid imbalance, or sickness and dis-ease.

This is why I am excited to introduce my beautiful and talented wife and her new and significant alkalizing recipe book. Shelley's recipes not only taste good, but also, they will energize and alkalize you from the inside out, keeping the internal alkaline fluids of the body balanced.

This recipe book will help guide you through the transition from an acid diet to eating alkaline food and enjoying every taste. I should know, because Shelley is my wife and she feeds me. I also know because I am a research scientist and I look at my blood on a regular basis. The blood is the river of life showing the state of imbalance or balance. So here are some pictures (shown below) of my balanced blood, energized and alkalized, by Shelley! Thank you, Shelley, for your inspiration and your dedica-tion, not only in helping me and our family stay energized and alkalized, but also for helping so many others return "Back to the House of Health."
All my love and support,

**Robert O. Young, Ph.D., D.Sc.**
*Husband, Father, and Scientist*

Healthy live blood

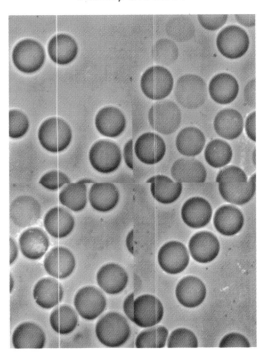

Healthy dried blood

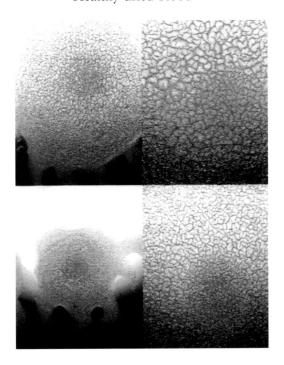

# *Preface*

There are millions of cookbooks out there in the world. Why would I feel it necessary to add one more? Because this recipe book is incredibly different! What makes it unique is the science that it is based upon: the "New Biology," as perceived and presented by my husband, Dr. Robert O. Young. At the basis of this healing science is the concept of alkalizing the pH of the blood and body tissues in order to create an environment (inner terrain) that is balanced and conducive to rejuvenation, healing, and wholeness.

I also know from my own background as a Licensed Massage Therapist the importance of the lymphatic system in handling and eliminating toxins from the body. This too must be kept in alkaline balance.

I trained as a microscopist for the Robert O. Young Research Testing Team and have observed thousands of blood samples from people all over the world. Over and over again I saw with my own eyes the changes, at the cellular level, that would occur when people made changes in their diet. As they adopted a more alkalizing diet, rich in raw vegetables, especially greens, I witnessed an extreme improvement in (1) red blood cell integrity, (2) oxygenation of the bloodstream, (3) diminishing yeast and fungal forms in the blood serum, and (4) a dramatic reduction in bacterial and higher pleomorphic and disturbing microforms found in the blood of sick and tired people!

As would be expected, I also witnessed the ultimate joy, smiles, relief, and renewed peace of mind from those who had turned a serious illness or symptomatology around to a state of balance—a return to the "House of Health," so to speak! People who were sick and tired got well and had energy again. They lost weight that they had been battling for years. Cholesterol levels dropped, skin cleared up, itching stopped, aches and pains disappeared, and in some extreme cases, insulin injections were no longer needed. People who had been diagnosed with cancer were pronounced cancer-free and tumors disappeared. People were so deeply grateful, and the same questions kept coming at me: What can I eat? How do you do this? How do I get my spouse and children to do this?

I knew that all of this healing occurred because people were willing to take the majority of the responsibility for their own health, and make the necessary CHANGE. They just weren't sure how to live the science continually from the kitchen, out in restaurants, and throughout their busy, fast-paced lifestyles. They also had been taught, through tradition and convenience, a lifestyle and way of eating that was extremely acidifying to the blood and tissues.

All one has to do is look around in any public place to see that people are suffering from obesity, fatigue, and premature aging. Almost all of us have a loved one who is suffering from one of the top three killers in the United States—heart disease, cancer, or diabetes. As one who watched her father lie on the couch for 12 years with Hodgkin's disease and the aftermath of chemotherapy and radiation, I felt there must be a better way and that there had to be a CHANGE!

This is why I decided to do yet another recipe book—one that guides a person through changing the pH of their blood and tissues from acid waste to alkaline balance, just by changing the way he/she arranges food on his/her plate. The book is also the solution to preserving variety, texture, and "out-of-this-world" flavors in breakfast, lunch, dinner, and ultra-healthy snacks. So eating alkaline becomes a gift we give ourselves, not a program of deprivation.

As you learn to eat 80 percent raw whole foods, and 20 percent warmed/cooked, grounding foods, your tastebuds will change. Your mental clarity may become sharper, and if you're like me, your body will thank you by functioning much more efficiently, so that you can have all that energy you thought was lost with your childhood.

I have always had a deep appreciation and respect for the foods that come from our Creator, from the land. I am totally convinced that it is in these "mostly green" alkalizing and energizing foods, or gifts, that a new millennium of healing can be ours, if we are just open and willing to accept an invitation to CHANGE.

**Shelley Redford Young**

# Acknowledgments

*Back to the House of Health* has been created from truly a partnership effort. It is a "culminate" form, evolved out of a "healing science" that was re-illuminated by my husband, Dr. Robert O. Young. There is no way I can adequately express my gratitude for him, his support, his dedication and perseverance in courageously bringing this truth and light to a suffering world. His contribution to mankind has made it possible for me to live out my most heartfelt desire—for people to be well, whole, and happy.

I also want to express my deepest appreciation for my sons, Adam, Andrew, and Alex and to my daughter, Ashley Rose. Thank you for listening and being patient, and for being open to the alkalizing healing message we share. You have all brought such great joy to my life!

I would like to thank our able editor, Jo Sinclair, for her patience, and for her great contributions that polished this work so it could shine. Also to Trent Tenney and Cord Udall at Woodland Publishing, whose efforts made the book possible in such a short time frame. Thanks for meeting the challenge.

Among dear friends whose support has been especially meaningful to this work, I want to include extended family members on both the Young and Redford sides, who have encouraged me to get a recipe book "out there" in the people's hands. You know who you are and I love you!

Also to the staff at Innerlight International, the Robert O. Young Research Center, the (blessed) Green Team, especially two angels of light, Shirley Dodd, and Jayna Catherine, and to the many microscopy students we have taught, who are truly satellites and take our message much further than we ever could alone. Thank you! Thank you!

To all of the true believers, Stu and Marybeth Mittleman, Russ and Mary Anne Green, and especially to Anthony Robbins for LAUNCHING our message in his wonderfully BIG rocket-ship way!

I am most grateful for the recipe contributions from some gracious healers: Angelique and Chrystyanna Queensley from Communication House, Salt Spring, BC, Canada, and also Maren Hale. Thank you for creating recipes that heal from the inside out!

To my two great assistants in the kitchen during the photography sessions, Jennifer Carpenter and Maren Hale, and to a dear friend, Jillair Meine, for the use of her lovely dishes, many thanks. Hey guys—with all our free time, let's start a cooly-cool vegan restaurant!

Finally to my photographer, Stefan Hallberg, thank you for demanding excellence, and for test-tasting every meal to make sure it was delicious (wink), and for presenting these gifts from God so beautifully.

In light and love,

*Shelley*

# *Introduction*

> *"Absorption and organization of sunlight, the very essence of life,
> is almost exclusively derived from plants. Plants are therefore
> a biological accumulation of light. Since light is the driving force of
> every cell in our bodies, that is why we need plants."*
>
> —Dr. Klinik Bircher-Benner

## An Invitation to Change

### What Can I Eat?

Congratulations! Your purchase of this alkalizing recipe book probably means you're preparing to embark on the adventure of a health-generating lifestyle. You may have heard Dr. Robert O. Young's science from a presentation or perhaps you have read his book, *Sick and Tired? Reclaim Your Inner Terrain,* and you want to know how to continually LIVE this science from the kitchen. Now, however, you open the fridge and cupboards and perhaps come to the GRIM reality that most of what is in there is very acid-forming or lacking in nutrition and fiber.

All food that is digested in our bodies metabolizes down to an ash residue. This ash residue can be neutral, acid, or alkaline. It is important to understand that the cells of our body are bathed in an alkaline fluid. Just as our body temperature is maintained at 98.6°F, our body fluids should be maintained at a 7.3–7.4 alkaline pH. Blood pH is ideally 7.365. Over-acidification of body fluids and tissues signals a state of imbalance, opening the door to sickness and disease. (As well, an overly alkaline blood pH signals a generally over-acidic condition, as the blood pulls in alkaline salts to neutralize the acidity.)

Foods which create an acid residue are meats and other flesh proteins, eggs, dairy products, yeast breads and yeast products, fermented foods (e.g., vinegar, soy sauce, miso, tempeh, sauerkraut, alcohol), sugars, and high-sugar

fruits. Dr. Young has found through scientific research that sugars, e.g., white sugar, brown sugar, maple syrup, high-fructose corn syrup, high-sugar fruits, fruit juice, and even high-sugar vegetables like carrots and beets, contribute to excess fermentation, which creates excess acidity in our body fluids. (Once a person becomes balanced, or symptom-free, the higher-sugar fruits can be eaten fresh and in season, occasionally, for cleansing purposes. But while symptoms of excess fermentation/acidity are present, they should be avoided.) As well, coffee, black tea, and soft drinks are highly acidifying.

Foods which create an alkaline residue are vegetables—especially greens of all kinds, such as spinach, cucumber, lettuce, grasses, celery, broccoli, etc.; soaked and sprouted seeds, nuts, and grains; and low-sugar fruits such as avocado, lemon, lime, tomato, and bell peppers. Raw foods are more alkalizing, while cooked food is more acidifying.

To maintain a balanced and alkalized pH in blood and tissues, the diet should contain at least 70–80 percent alkalizing foods, and no more than 20–30 percent cooked or acidifying foods.

Our bodies are similar to our Earth, which is 70 percent water with 30 percent mass. Therefore it makes

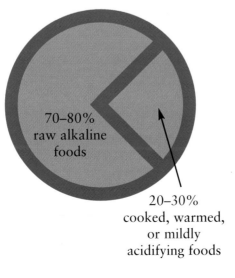

70–80%
raw alkaline
foods

20–30%
cooked, warmed,
or mildly
acidifying foods

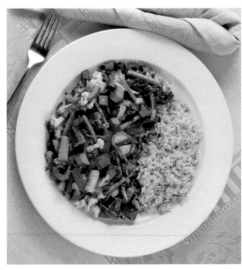

sense to keep our meals based in high-water content foods that are alkalizing to the blood and tissues.

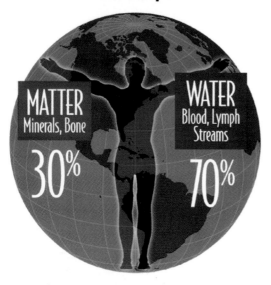

Our bodies also break down to :

70% water
1–2% vitamins and minerals
1/2–1% sugar
20% fat
7% protein

The recipes in this book are designed with a similar breakdown, to help you arrange balanced alkalizing meals and return to your House of Health. Recipes that require no cooking (in other words, recipes that are "raw") are called FOUNDATIONAL, which means they are 100% alkalizing. These should be used when a person is on the cleanse phase of Dr. Young's Complete Program and Diet™ (contact the Robert O. Young Research Center at 801-756-7850 for information), or when dealing with any specific or serious symptomatology or imbalance. Once a person feels balanced and is no longer dealing with symptoms, the rest of the recipes, which I call FRAMEWORK recipes, could then be used, maintaing a balance of 80 percent alkalizing and 20 percent acidifying visual arrangement on the plate. An example would be a nice big salad with a side of the baked Tofu Italian Mock Meatballs and Roasted Bell Pepper Sauce.

To supplement the diet, I have also included the ROOF recipes. These would include healthy alkalizing snacks, like raw almond butter on sprouted wheat tortillas, perfect for those times when you just need a quick bite or for children who almost live on snacks.

Moving towards an alkalizing lifestyle and diet is a process—not an overnight event. So when you make the decision to come back to the House of Health, enjoy your journey home. During this journey, changes may occur. Tastebuds that have been jaded by the toxic effect of extreme sugars and salt, may take some time to appreciate the subtler and humbler sweetness of vegetables. Sometimes people experience some cleansing symptoms such as headaches, fatigue, lightheadedness, rash, or bad breath, as the body literally cleans house and gets rid of toxins that have been stored in the tissues and bloodstream. Through phasing and transition (see Chapter 1), one can make this CHANGE an exciting, rewarding gift that is pro-active and lasting in your life. It may be a welcome surprise to find how quick, easy, economical, and tasty the arranged alkalizing meals can be. Happy Healing! Bon Appetit!

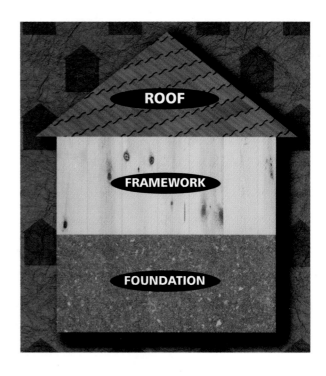

# The Basics

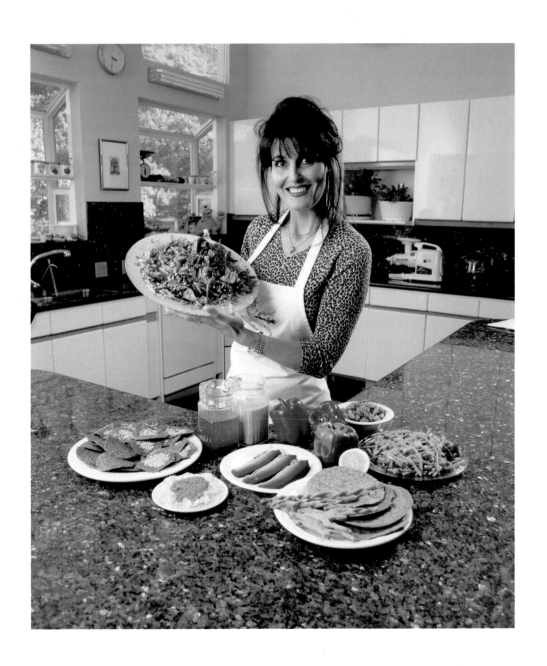

## Why Alkalize?

Dr. Young teaches that sugar, yeast, starch, and animal foods are the ones that morbid pleomorphic microforms live and multiply on, creating mycotoxins (fungal poisons) that are designed to decompose us and which leave us sick and tired! (Refer to his book, *Sick and Tired? Reclaim Your Inner Terrain.*) Let's consider some recent statistics:

- One in eight school children has high blood pressure.
- Four to six children in 30 are on some type of drug for Attention Deficit Disorder.
- Children are on the average 12 lb. heavier than they were 20 years ago.
- Half of us will die from heart disease or diabetes.
- One-third of us will die from cancer.
- 24 million suffer from insomnia.
- 55 million suffer from regular recurring headaches.
- 15 million are alcoholics.
- 60% of us are overweight.
- 15 million suffer from disastrous side-effects from prescription drugs.

When I was in junior high school and my father came down with cancer, there were two of us in a class of 30 that had a family member with this serious disease. Now when I lecture to audiences and ask how many of them have a family member suffering from one of the top three killers—cancer, heart disease, or diabetes—70–80 percent of the audience raise their hands. Something needs to change. And we have to realize once and for all that there is NO magic bullet. The Phen-fen (diet pill) fiasco is a perfect example of this: Women wishing to lose weight ended up with heart valve damage.

The USDA food pyramid currently taught in the schools is quite behind in teaching alkalizing principles to our youth. Let's review what is currently being taught and supported by the USDA food pyramid and compare that to Dr. Young's pyramid.

The USDA food pyramid metabolizes down to a high amount of sugar from complex and simple carbohydrates—from pasta and grains at the base, from fruits in the second step, milk products (lactose) in the third step, and from sweets at the top. Also, meat and other flesh foods in the third step contribute to acidity. Therefore the USDA food pyramid is a highly acidifying food plan.

Dr. Young's food pyramid promotes alkalinity of the blood and tissues by basing the diet around alka-lizing vegetables, sprouted and soaked nuts and seeds, essential oils, and low-sugar fruits. An emphasis on "greens" also supplies us with chlorophyll, which is molecularly structured like our own hemoglobin. Dr. Young's pyramid is alkalizing and sup-

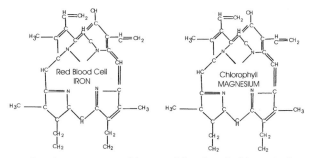

**Molecular structure of human blood and chlorophyll**

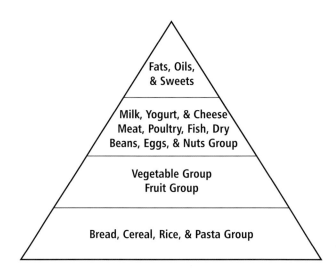

## USDA Food Pyramid (acid forming)

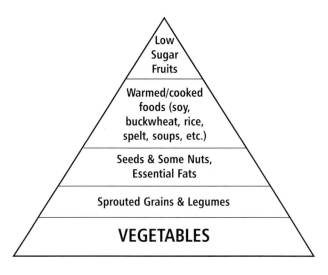

## Dr. Young's Pyramid (alkaline forming)

portive for balancing the pH of the blood and tissues in our bodies. (See *Sick and Tired? Reclaim Your Inner Terrain,* Chapter 5, for further information on acid/alkaline balance.)

Remember that when you build an alkalizing meal, raw vegetables are going to be the most alkalizing and energy-packed (life-force) foods you can eat. As Dr. Klinik Bircher-Benner has said, "The closer food is to the natural sun energy, the higher it is in all levels of nutritional value for the human organism."

## The Protein/Calcium Myth

Two of the most common questions we are asked are: "Where do you get your protein?" and "What about calcium?" It is evident that most people think protein and calcium need to come from meat and dairy products to be complete. This simply is not so. Formerly, vegetable proteins were classified as second class, but this distinction has now been generally discarded. Why? Because vegetables carry the sub-cellular units (microzymas) and the amino acids to make proteins. Also, all green vegetables are high in calcium. From observing some of the strongest animals in the world, who mostly graze on grasses, we see that they are getting plenty of protein and calcium. Whenever we are asked where we get our protein and calcium, we reply, "Where does the cow get hers?"

We have to evaluate just how much protein we really need. Again, our bodies break down to 70 percent water, 1–2 percent vitamins and minerals, 0.5–1 percent sugar, 20 percent fat, and 7 percent protein. Human mother's milk is only 5 percent protein, or some sources state as little as 1.4–2.2 percent. A newborn's growth demand is to double or triple body mass and size within the first year of life. One would think, if protein were needed in such high quantity for good growth and health, that mother's milk would contain a much higher percentage, but it doesn't!

The high-protein approach to nutrition was initially based on 19th century German research which said that humans needed a minimum of 120 grams of protein per day. Conventional nutritionists dropped this to 60 to 90 grams a day, and more recently, expert research suggests closer to 25 grams a day. Consider the following clinical study reported in the *Journal of the American Dietetic Association.* This study compared the essential amino acids in the diets of meat-eaters, lacto-ovo vegetarians (those who eat dairy and eggs), and pure vegan vegetarians. The study uncompromisingly set the protein requirements for each amino acid at the level that would easily cover the needs of growing children and pregnant women. The results? Not only did ALL three diets provide sufficient protein, they were all WELL ABOVE sufficient, each diet exceeding twice its requirement!!

Another U.S. journal reported the following: The average American meat-eater consumes one-and-a-half to four times more protein than is really needed. According to many scientists, this is the main reason for osteoporosis, the bone-weakening disease that strikes 45,000 American women each year. When you eat too many acidic meat and dairy proteins, your blood tries to return to its alkaline state the only way it can—by withdrawing calcium from your bones. The irony is that even if you're eating plenty of calcium-rich foods, you can have a negative calcium balance and an increased risk of osteoporosis! Your kidneys also rob your bones in order to eliminate the excess nitrogen found in animal protein. This research should lead us to stop worrying about getting enough protein and raise the concern about whether we are actually getting too much.

There is also a correlation between cancer and high-protein intake. From Dr. T. Colin Campbell, director of the Division of Nutritional Sciences at Cornell University and former senior science advisor to the American Institute for Cancer Research, we read the following:

*There is a strong correlation between dietary protein intake and cancer of the breast, prostate, pancreas, and colon. The culprit in many of the most prevalent and deadly diseases of our time, according to this study, is none other than the very thing many of us have been taught to hold virtually sacred—animal protein. People who derive 70% of their protein from animal products have major health difficulties compared to people who derive just 5% of their protein from animal sources. They have 17 times the death rate from heart disease and the women are 5 times more likely to die of breast cancer. In conclusion, animal protein is at the core of many chronic diseases.*

Most meats are 20–25 percent protein. Eating meat can give us protein; however, along with this protein comes saturated fat and possible synthetic hormones, steroids and antibiotics that have been given to the animal. Also, pesticide chemicals can be in the meat from the grain fed to the animal. Along with all of this, morbid pathogenic bacteria loads from the fermentation of acids can be present in the animal tissues, before or at the time of slaughter.

And a note about "protein combining." The recognition that many fruits, vegetables, grasses, legumes and grains fall short in certain amino acids led to the development of the complementary protein principle, in vogue for many years. For example, grains are low in the essential amino acid lysine. Legumes, or beans, are low in another amino acid, methionine. By combining the two foods one supplies the lacking or limited amino acids, thereby improving both foods' biological value. Thus the combining of foods was thought to be necessary because all essential amino acids must be present for protein synthesis to occur in the body.

What this idea overlooked was that the body has a free amino acid pool, a constantly changing supply of amino acids derived from body sources, as cells that were once organized, like red blood cells, disorganize to provide microzymas, which then organize themselves into protein complexes. This body pool contributes about 70 grams of protein daily. Thus, the idea that you need to eat all the essential amino acids simultaneously is erroneous. In reality, all you need are those tiny, indestructible, intelligent beings—the microzymas—found in all green foods.

Now that we've taken a serious look at the protein/calcium myth that exits, let's now look at the percentage of protein calories derived from vegetables and other vegan foods:

| | |
|---|---|
| Spinach | 49% |
| Broccoli | 47% |
| Tofu | 43% |
| Green Leaf Lettuce | 42% |
| Alfalfa Sprouts | 40% |
| Kale | 40% |
| Lentils | 30% |
| Green Peas | 30% |
| Zucchini | 26% |
| Navy Beans | 26% |
| Wheat Grass | 25% |
| Garbanzo Beans | 25% |
| Garlic | 20% |
| Pumpkin Seeds | 20% |
| Tomatoes | 18% |
| Sunflower Seeds | 17% |
| Sprouted Sunflower Seeds | 33% |
| Wheat | 17% |
| Avocado | 15% |
| Almonds | 15% |
| Lemons | 13% |

Again, there seems to be a general opinion out in the public that eating a vegan diet would seriously deplete one's calcium intake, which is vital for so many functions of the body. Many commercials promote dairy foods and even antacids (Tums®) as a way to get our required daily percentage of calcium. Some of these commercials target women and use osteoporosis as a reason to take their products or supplements. The fact is, ALL green leafy vegetables and grasses are inherently HIGH in calcium, iron, magnesium, vitamin C, and many of the B vitamins. These would include: all grasses, spinach, parsley, cabbage, kale, collard greens, celery, cauliflower, beet greens, green leafy lettuce, okra, onions, green beans. Also, avocado, black beans, garbanzo beans, tofu, almonds, hazelnuts, and sesame seeds are all very high in calcium. Again ask yourself, Where does the cow get her calcium? As long as we are eating an alkalizing diet that is rich in green foods and green drinks, we don't need to worry about getting enough calcium.

Dr. Young and I recently had a bone density test to determine if we had any signs of calcium deficiency. We have been vegans for approximately 20 years now, and both of our tests came out with bone densities that were well above average. My rating was similar to a 20-year-old's bone density (I am 46). Dr. Young's was also in the very highest percentage; he is 48.

# Phasing and Transition

## Shaping Your Approach

Now come the questions: How do I do this? How can I alkalize my bloodstream? How do I cook? How do I get my spouse and family to do this? How do I eat at a restaurant? Will this really help me? And the all-time winner: What can I eat?

To make this change we must first have an awareness—such as, "Whoa! I'm getting fat!" Or, "I really don't feel like I used to." Or, "I'm sick and I don't want to be this way anymore!"—that moves us to investigation. Hopefully, after hearing the InnerLight science, the New Biology, and the research behind it, we can develop understanding or knowledge about what we have heard and seen. Once we can see the potential this science and alkalizing diet have in our lives or in that of a loved one who is suffering, we can then move to action and, with patience, get the results we desire. The process goes: Awareness, Investigation, Knowledge, Potential, Motivation, Action, Patience, Results.

There is also another order in the process that can work for some people who don't feel they know, but still have a desire to find out. With this attitude: "Well, I don't know that all this is true, but I think I'll give it a try, just to see," you could start with action, i.e., the alkalizing diet. Then if you start to get results, this will create confidence that the diet works, which will carry you on to recognizing the potential, and move you to more committed action, patience, and more results.

## Motivation is Key

Commitment, which is an aspect of motivation, is vital. W.H. Murray brilliantly describes the support that can arise when one is committed:

*Until one is committed, there is hesitancy, the chance to draw back, always ineffectiveness. Concerning all acts of initiative (and creation) there is one elementary truth, the ignorance of which kills countless ideas and splendid plans: that the moment one commits oneself, then Providence moves too. All sorts of things occur to help one that otherwise would never have occurred. A whole stream of events issues from the decision, raising in one's favor all manner of unforeseen incidents and meetings and material assistance, which no man could have dreamt would have come his way.*

I have learned a deep respect for one of Goethe's couplets: *"Whatever you can do or dream you can, begin it. Boldness has genius, power and magic in it."*

### 1. Record your motivation.

The first step in focusing on your motivation is to state the change you want to see in your life, and then write it down in the form of a desired outcome; e.g., "I want to be free of my headaches so I can enjoy more activities with my family;" or, "I want to be slim again;" or, "I want to be well again."

### 2. Set a realistic and appropriate plan, including a time frame.

It is wise to be very realistic and plan for what we know we can do. However, this will depend on your motivation, your desired outcome, and your condition. The more imbalanced or sick a person is, the more reason to find the motivation, and the more commitment is required to find balance and wholeness. It will not profit someone who is seriously ill to say, for example, "I'll go off hard sugars, but I just can't give up my sourdough bread and fruit!" If you were to think of the balanced state as the House of Health, then we would have to agree that if you are very far from home you won't be able to return by

going only half-way back. If garbage attracts flies, you can't get rid of the flies by taking out half the garbage, right?

A realistic plan: "I will take the next six months to do all I can to eliminate my headaches. I will go on Dr. Young's Complete Program and Diet™ (contact the Robert O. Young Research Center at 801-756-7850), drink green juices, and make dietary changes that will help bring my body into a state of balance."

### 3. Avoid extremes (unless you are acutely sick).

Once you have decided what your motivation is, break each new behavior change down into steps, so that reclaiming your terrain becomes an exciting process, not an overwhelming, overnight challenge. Introduce new healthy habits into your daily routine by making statements like: "I will start drinking fresh vegetable juices and add them to my diet at least three times a week." Or, "I will start drinking one glass of concentrated green juice once a day. Also, I will start by going off hard sugars for one week, and then phase out the high-sugar fruits until I reach a state of proper balance."

### 4. Practice your new habits.

Practice having a totally alkaline breakfast at least five times a week, then extend that to seven days a week. Instead of thinking, "You deserve a break today, so get up and get away to McDonald's," the thinking has to change to "You (your blood and tissues) really deserve a break from all that acidity today, so get up and stay away from McDonald's."

Practice going without a heavy, sugary dessert after dinner. Practice skipping the alcoholic beverage before dinner. Practice choosing a vegetarian entrée in the restaurant. Practice is repetition, and we know that repetition of any skill will increase our ability in that skill. As you practice these new, healthy habits, you will develop a skilled, intuitive way of feeding your body what it needs without feelings of deprivation. Instead of thinking about what you can't have, you will begin to look forward to the fresh green salad you are blessed to have. The journey Back to the House of Health can become one of the greatest and most abundant gifts you give to that very important person—YOU!

### 5. Evaluate, review, and reward your progress.

Closely monitor your symptoms. Are they diminishing, or have they gone? Do you feel lighter, brighter, more energetic? Have you lost some weight? Do your clothes fit better? Ask yourself,

"Did I stay alkaline most of the month?" If you are unable to make the desired change at first, then re-evaluate your goal. If you see that it is too harsh, adjust it (within the bounds of appropriateness to your condition) so that it is more reasonable for you to achieve.

Actually the best reward for bringing your body into balance could simply be the disappearance of symptoms, but if you feel you need other rewards, make the rewards non-food items, like a new pair of pants. Or treat yourself to a class you've always wanted to take. Buy a piece of art and hang it in your home for a reward.

At this point we need to remind you that sometimes you can get worse before you get better. When we embark on a healthful regime, there can (but not always) be cleansing symptoms such as rash, bad breath, headaches, weakness, and fatigue while the body is adjusting and dealing with the stirring up and surfacing of toxins that are coming out of tissues. (One word on rashes or other skin reactions—do not suppress them with drugs or medications. At most use pure moisturizer or liquid vitamin E.) If given a chance and some patience and time, the body can be a great house-cleaner and rebuilder. Also, expect some adjustments in tastebuds, which have been saturated with sweet and salty food for years. Eventually, vegetables will taste sweet, and a cookie or a candy bar may become too sweet, even intolerable. There may also be some cravings until addictions wear off and blood sugar levels stabilize. Understanding why these situations arise will help you stay with the program and complete the transition phase that comes with change.

**6. If you "fall off the wagon" or "eat too acid" one day, simply go forward.**

Feeling guilty or down about your mistake is a waste of time and a drain of energy. Forgive yourself and just get back on the wagon: Restate your motivation and goals. Once you arrive at your House of Health, an occasional outing may not be very harmful, keeping Home in view and not straying very far from the truths you've acquired.

When we consider these steps to introducing change, there are some ideas that have helped us and our family with the transitions.

## Transition 1: Breakfast

The most common questions we're asked by people who are changing their life and their diet are, "What can I eat?" and "How do I cook or prepare food?"

First, there must be a change of heart and mind concerning breakfast. Most American or European breakfast foods are problematic and predispose the body to infectious and degenerative symptoms. Foods such as cereals, sweet rolls, toast, pancakes, waffles, muffins, oatmeal, maple syrup, honey, orange juice, etc., are too high in sugars and carbohydrates, which over-acidify the blood and tissues. Any excess sugar not converted to energy in the blood is stored as fat in the fat cells. This is the reason why many people are fat, sick, and tired! High-protein, high-fat, acidifying breakfast foods such as dairy, eggs, sausage, bacon, etc., also compromise the biological terrain and ultimately promote the growth of morbidly evolved bacteria, yeast, fungus, and mold. What is worse, many of these substances are eaten in combinations which disrupt digestion, resulting in fermentation and putrefaction. By the way, about 20 minutes after eating an egg, a person will show a presence or high increase of bacteria in their blood.

Vegetable soup is a great way to start the day! In the late 18th century, an all-night taverner named Boulanger began selling soups which he called "restoratives" or "restorantes" to weary travelers. Boulanger is not only credited with creating the birth of the restaurant profession, his creativity with soups led to their popularity in France. Hearty soups and stews course through the body with a good glow that lasts for hours. Other breakfast choices for us include: a glass of fresh vegetable juice or a fresh green salad with plenty of different sprouts, garnished with flax seed oil, lemon, and Bragg™ Liquid Aminos. Sometimes we have a bowl of basmati rice, topped with fresh avocado, tomato, spouts, soaked almonds, and a seasoning called "The Zip" by Spice Hunter. We also add some good oil, lemon or lime juice, and Liquid Aminos, too. Also, veggie wraps are a great start to the day: we wrap up a bunch of fresh or steamed vegetables, soaked seeds, and a few sun-dried tomatoes in a sprouted wheat tortilla. Yum!

## Transition 2: Breakfast, Lunch, and Dinner Become Synonymous as a Time to Nourish and Rebuild

Any meal you build should stay at least in a 70 percent alkaline to 30 percent acid ratio. Better yet, an 80 percent to 20 percent ratio, especially if you are ill. With this in mind, a given combination can usually be eaten for breakfast, lunch, or dinner. This is not universally true since it has been found that a particular food might sit very well with someone at one time of day, but not another. Other exceptions may arise from a number of factors, such as activity level, biochemical makeup, or closeness of the last meal to bedtime, for example. You will gradually learn what works for you. Some dietary approaches suggest making lunch the biggest meal, while eating lightly at supper. There is some merit to this, especially if supper tends to be later in the evening, closer to bedtime. Never forget, however, that you are unique, and that any "perfect" program is there to give you a foundation. From there, finding what works for you involves taking personal responsibility.

## Transition 3: Condiments

Most condiments are acid-forming. Catsup, mustard, vinegar, sugars, soy sauces, cream sauces, etc., contain fermented and highly acidifying ingredients. If you had a child who was going around with the type of friends that were having a bad influence on him/her, what would your greatest wish for your child be? To make new friends, of course! You probably need to make new friends and give up old friends in the condiments category.

Here are our new condiment friends:

- *Bragg™ Liquid Aminos.*
- *Good oils:* The oils we have found to be best are borage oil, flax seed oil, marine lipids, pumpkin, and olive oil. (Put oil on food after cooking so you don't change the fatty acid chains.) One salad dressing we suggest is Annie's Naturals Organic Green Garlic.
- *Lemon:* Lemon is a great low-sugar fruit that adds freshness and zest to many dishes (when used in proper food combination, described below). It can be used as a sugar-crave buster and blood alkalizer, and is high in vitamin C.
- *Spices:* Get creative with spices, but don't abuse them. "The Zip" by Spice Hunter is a great, tangy spice containing onion, paprika, chili pepper, cumin, garlic, jalapeño, coriander, cayenne, and oregano. Spice Hunter takes a lot of the guesswork out of spicing your dishes, and has a wonderful inventory of creative combinations. Experiment! Most health food stores carry Spice Hunter spices, but they may be difficult to find in some areas. Their toll-free number is 800-444-3061.
- *Garlic, Onion, Ginger:* These are all naturally anti-fungal and anti-parasitical.

## Transition 4: Phasing

It took over a year for us to phase milk, risen bread, and meat out of our kitchen. If you want to eat animal protein, our recommendation would be to cook trout or salmon, as we feel they are the best choices because of their omega 3 (essential fatty acid) content.

To phase out risen bread, we went to yeast-free bread, then rice crackers, then whole wheat sprouted tortillas and cooked grains like millet, spelt, rice, buckwheat. Soba noodles are also a favorite in our home and satisfy the need for a chewy, warm food, especially in winter. Remember to keep most grains in your 20 percent acid part of your meal. (Buckwheat and spelt are not acidifying.)

To phase out meat, we went from no red meat or chicken, to turkey, to fish, to tofu, to raw almonds, hazelnuts, and seeds like raw sunflower, pumpkin, flax, and sesame. Soak nuts and seeds overnight if possible, as this activates enzymes and increases nutrition. Almonds are especially good; they are substantially alkalizing and high in protein and calcium. Wheat grass and other greens such as spinach carry a higher amino acid count than steak!

To phase out dairy (milk and cheese), we went from milk to soy milk, to Rice Dream®, to fresh vegetable juices.

To phase out sugary desserts we went from ice-cream and baked desserts to frozen yogurt, to Rice Dream® bars, to fresh fruit, to veggies! Now a treat for us is a crisp, red bell pepper or thick slices of jicama, which is a tasty root vegetable of low-sugar, high-water content that tastes like a cross between an apple and potato. For the most part we don't do dessert. On vacation we break down once in a while, only when we feel we are balanced and well; then we get right back to 80 percent alkaline and 20 percent acid the very next day.

## Transition 5: Crunchies and Munchies

To deal with the need for something to chew and crunch on, we went from cookies and corn chips to brown rice crackers, baked sprouted tortillas, raw almonds (best soaked), and raw veggies. Also baked (fresh) tofu is a snack in our house. Again, one of our favorite crunchies is jicama. Sliced cold it's a great treat to crunch on and helps during sugar cravings.

## Transition 6: Socializing and Going to Restaurants

Restaurants are beginning to "come around" in that a lot of them offer vegetarian entrées. If you stick with Asian and Chinese you're fairly safe. Also, most restaurants have side salads or dishes that could be ordered to build a meal from (a green dinner salad, a side of fresh veggies, with a side of beans or rice or baked potato makes a pretty good meal). Also, don't be afraid to make requests. We do it all the time to avoid mushrooms, for example. Most chefs are happy to do a stir-fry if you request it.

If you are traveling, look in the phone book. In most places you can find a health food store or vegetarian restaurant. While in New York, we were able to make a beautiful alkaline meal in any of the corner delis, and most of them did fresh juicing.

The value of change is in the result, and in realizing the peace and harmony that arise from embracing the change as part of everyday behavior. It's in wanting the very best for ourselves and those we love, and being willing to examine and understand the information and truths coming out of the research. It's in being whole and strong so we can help someone else who needs to make this change.

# Food Combining for Digestion

There are many food combining charts on the market, suggesting different points of view which can be very confusing and inaccurate. For example, they may say lemons, limes and tomatoes are acid-producing and should not be combined with starches or proteins. Another example would be that avocados are a protein fruit and should not be combined with starches or proteins. Both of these examples do not consider the fact that the first thing that ferments in any organized matter, once it has been disturbed by chewing, is the sugar. That is, the tiny intelligent indestructible beings (microzymas) that make up that matter move from respiration to sugar metabolism as the matter breaks down (digests). Because lemons, limes, tomatoes and avocados are low-sugar/high-water content fruits, they produce very little acid residue and are highly alkalizing. The key to good digestion is not how we combine foods but how we choose foods to eat which are most like us: high water (70% or greater), naturally occurring oils (20–30%), low protein (5–7%), and even lower sugar (0.5 to 3%). Understanding that our bodies are a gelatinous (between a liquid and a solid) material

in an ocean of water, we do not have to worry ourselves with food combining ideologies or charts when we are eating high-water/low-sugar content foods! This is important to understand, since the water and sugar content of each food we organize into a meal becomes the most important indicator for food combination, rather than whether the food is a vegetable, fruit, or protein.

There are several fundamental rules in food combining that are very important and not understood by many savants and nutritionists. They include:

1. All high-sugar fruits are acid-forming and should not be combined with other types of foods or ingested in a state of imbalance; e.g., bananas (25% sugar), apples (15%), oranges (12%), mangoes (18%), pineapples (28%), strawberries (11%), cherries (12%), watermelon (9%), and honeydew (21%).
2. Low-sugar fruits are alkalizing and can be combined with vegetables or proteins, e.g. avocado (2% sugar), tomato (3%), lemon (3%), lime (3%), cantaloupe (5 %), and non-sweet grapefruit (5%).
3. Low-sugar/high-water fruits and vegetables can be combined with each other or with proteins or starches.
4. If in a state of imbalance, go easy on the high-sugar vegetables, e.g., carrots (11% sugar), beets (13%), and high-sugar squash. Although carrot itself is an alkalizing vegetable, if taken in excess, as concentrated carrot juice, the sugar content is too high. (Acids are produced by morbid fermentation of sugar.)
5. Cold-pressed, polyunsaturated fats (flax seed oil, borage oil, marine lipids, evening primrose oil), monounsaturated fats (olive oil, avocado), and saturated fats (avocado) can be combined with vegetables, some fruits (lemons, limes, tomatoes, avocados, bell peppers), starches and vegetable proteins.

The outline below covers the basics of how to combine foods.

## The Basics of Combining

1. **Eat low-sugar/high-water vegetables or fruits with:**

   A. *Plant or animal protein.*
   B. *Starch.*
   C. *Cold-pressed oils.*

2. **Don't eat animal protein (this does not apply to vegetable or fruit protein) with:**

A. *Starch.* Animal protein digests in the stomach producing an acid medium (uric acid). When starch is combined with animal protein, the sugars in the starch create even more acid (acetic acid), leading to indigestion, heartburn and gas.

B. *Acids.* The digestion of food is a process of fermentation which gives rise to waste products known as acids or ferments. High-sugar fruits (which are highly acid-producing) accompanying animal protein increase the production of ferments in the stomach, giving rise to indigestion, heartburn and gas. Exception: Seeds, nuts and avocado (excellent sources of good fat) can be combined with plant or animal protein, starches, or high-sugar fruits.

C. *Oils.* Cold-pressed oils are essential for the construction of cell membranes, the production of hormones, and the chelation of acids or ferments. They can be eaten liberally with vegetable meals. However, with animal protein, oils will slow down the fermentation process (due to their chelating effect on the acids produced), causing congestion (constipation), which when piled up with other foods, especially fruits and carbohydrates, will create morbid mass leading to acid reflux, heartburn and gas.

3. **Don't eat starches (including starchy vegetables) with:**

A. *Animal protein.* Meat and potatoes is a perfect combination for indigestion.

B. *Acids, such as vinegar.* (In fact never ever eat vinegar; it is poisonous.) Acids mask the presence of starch in the mouth and block the action of ptyalin, a necessary component of starch digestion in saliva.

C. *High-sugar fruit.* High-sugar fruits like apples, oranges and bananas create excess acidity in the blood and poison the immune system, shutting it down for up to five hours. When you add starches like potatoes, bread, or pasta to the brew, you have sugar on top of sugar, or more acid on top of more acid, and the immune system is paralyzed for even longer periods of time. Note: Avocado (low-sugar/high-protein fruit) combines well with starches, e.g. grains, legumes, and starchy vegetables like yams.

D. *Oil.* Oil slows digestion of starch due to its chelating effect on the acids produced as the starch (sugar) ferments. However, this is not a problem if you keep at least 80% of the rest of the meal high-water/low-sugar content (i.e., plenty of veggies).

4. **Don't eat fruit* with:**

A. *Protein.* Obvious reasons. A fruit salad with a steak is a recipe for excess acid, leading to indigestion and gas. Exception: Fruit can be combined with avocado (low-sugar/protein fruit).

B. *Starch.* It's a taste temptation, like a peanut butter and banana sandwich (except if you think about a lemon sandwich!), but just too much difference here in digestion time (fruit digests quickly), so the combination begs for fermentation. However, the main thing that makes this combination so tempting to begin with is its added sugar (jam on toast, for example), and this makes the whole deal much worse.

C. *Vegetables.* Fruits are cleansers, veggies are builders. Don't ask the body to do opposites simultaneously. Exception: tomato, avocado, lemon and lime combine with all veggies.

D. *Oil.*

*Don't use fruit at all (except lemon, lime, raw tomato, avocado, and non-sweet grapefruit) until you are well, and then in moderation and in season.*

5. **Oils.**

Combine best with vegetables and fresh veggie juices; combine poorly with fruits (except tomato, avocado, lemon and lime).

6. **Melons.**

Eat melons alone, or not at all. Best to avoid them altogether, as they are very high in sugar (except cantaloupe), which means more acid. Also, like grapes and a few other sugary fruits, they can be high in mold. Once you are well and strong, an occasional treat is fine.

If you are seriously ill, or interested in following an ideal regimen, food combining is essential, as is the proper ratio of raw foods. Try taking smaller bites of food to enhance digestion through more chewing. Above all, don't discourage yourself by trying to change too much too quickly. Making gradual dietary changes is generally best for the body anyway. The exception to this might be when serious illness threatens your life or promises to inflict permanent damage. At such times, drastic change may do very nicely! The human digestive system is not designed for complex meals. It's best not to mix more than four foods, or food from more than two classes. Use only one protein per meal. And when you start using complex starches, only one per meal also.

Be careful not to wash food down with beverages, especially cold ones, including cold water. Cold shuts down digestive activity as easily as it preserves food. Because water dilutes digestive chemicals, it should be drunk at least a half-hour before, or one hour after, a meal which includes animal protein. But if you are eating a low-sugar/high-water content vegetarian meal, feel free to drink with your meal. It is helpful to eat juicier food items (veggies/salads) first to pave the way for heavier items. A few sips of warm water after a meal can aid digestion.

## A Few Special Notes

As mentioned, tomato is not a vegetable. It is a fruit, and as long as it is eaten raw, it is alkaline-forming, because of its low-sugar content. (When cooked it becomes acid-forming, though moderately so.) Low-sugar fruits and vegetables do combine, whereas high-sugar fruits and vegetables do not. Recipes with vegetables, starches, or proteins can be improved immensely by including the tomato, or avocado. Fresh tomato and basil on pasta with lots of olive oil is an excellent combination. Similarly, lemon juice can be used in dressings and included with starch, proteins, or oils. This avoids the dangers of vinegar and is an excellent substitution.

Avocado is a low-sugar/protein/fat fruit. It will combine with vegetables, even the starchy ones, and it will combine with grains, or with low- or high-sugar fruit. For example: avocado sandwich on yeast-free spelt bread, or avocado and tomato slices with lemon juice on jasmine rice.

Use liberal amounts of good oil with vegetable meals—flax seed oil, olive oil, borage oil, or a combination like Udo's Choice® found in your local health food store—to protect the body from acid wastes. Don't heat oils! Add a spoonful of oil to vegetables after warming or steaming. A flavorful salad dressing can be made with any of these oils combined with lemon and Bragg™ Liquid Aminos or yeast-free seasoning of your choice.

In general, apply heat gently and in moderation.

Avoid the burning, crisping and browning that frequently converts food into toxins. It is best to steam food or cook lightly in a small amount of water. Use moderate heat not to exceed 118°F. Another option is to use a non-stick cooking spray, made of lecithin. Some recipes may need a little experimentation on your part to come out "just right."

Make sure all foods and seasonings are yeast free.

## Getting Started: The Proper Tools

### Tools and Equipment

It is possible to arrange alkalizing meals with just one good knife and plenty of time; however, as any good carpenter knows, the proper tools do the job faster, easier, and with optimum results. You can always start out with an inexpensive food processor and blender to get yourself going on this great alkalizing lifestyle change. Then as you permanently change to an alkalizing diet, you can ask for BIG-ticket kitchen appliance tools for Christmas or your birthday! Or you can just invest in them as you are able to.

Below are the kitchen tools I find best suit me.

**GOOD KNIVES** are a must, since raw veggies need to be cleaned, cut, chopped, or trimmed most of the time. I love Cutco® knives with the bowling ball-material handles that are shaped to fit your hand grip. I started out with a three-piece starter set which included a short straight-edged paring knife, a longer serrated knife, and a serrated spatula spreader knife. I used this and got along quite well for years before investing in a larger set.

A **FOOD PROCESSOR** will cut your chopping, blending, and mixing time by as much as 90 percent, especially when you are preparing food for many people. I use the Cuisinart® brand, and started with the 7-cup size. When I started preparing food for large crowds, I invested in the 16-cup size. This food processor comes with both a sharp and soft-edged S-blade. I use these for almost all my chopping and mixing needs. I use the soft-edged S-blade to mix the dough for tortillas, and the sharp S-blade for mincing, fine and coarse chopping, and super-blending for foods like hummus or salad dressings, where ingredients must be emulsified for a smooth result. Along with the S-blades, the Cuisinart® also comes with shredding and slicing wheels, which I use to make beautiful salads. You can

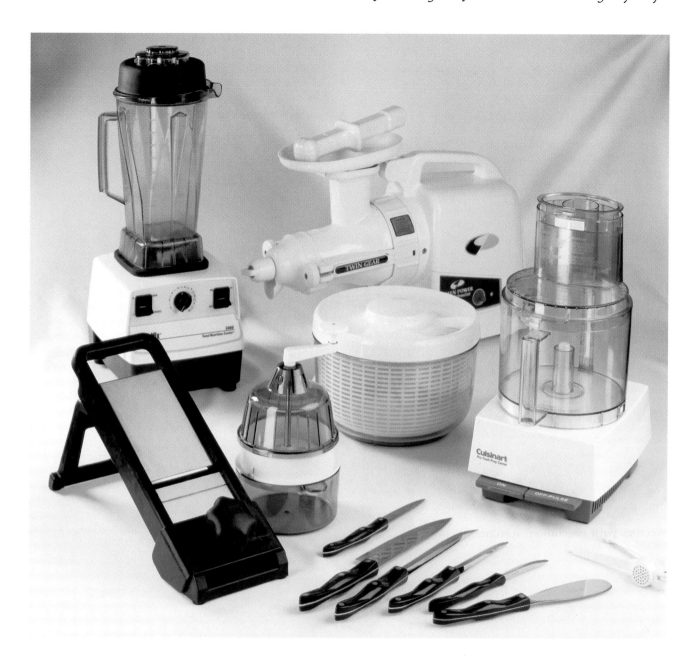

also grind dry ingredients like nuts and dried tortillas into powders in the Cuisinart®.

The **BLENDER** I prefer is the Vita-Mix®. The motor is very strong and has a good variety of options for speed control, and a reverse option. This blender also warms food while you blend, so recipes like the raw soups can be worked up very fast and served immediately straight from the blender. The Vita-Mix® is also able to grind dry ingredients, such as grains, seeds and nuts, and even mix dough.

I prefer the Green Power® **JUICER** for fresh juicing, mainly because it is one of the only juicers that will do grasses along with all other vegetables. A magnetic process also ionizes the juice. I keep mine right alongside the disposal side of the sink to catch the pulp. This is a rotary-geared machine that grinds the vegetables and then has a gravity fall for the juice (versus a centrifugal spinning juicer that needs the filter changed). It also comes with attachments for pasta and baby-food processing. What a great way to take your alkalizing meal and make it palatable for junior!

I keep a **RICE COOKER** on the counter, full of freshly steamed rice or other grain for the family to help themselves to any time during the day. I like the Zojirushi® brand, which will also cook legumes. This is a great thing to have on hand to build the 20–30 percent more grounding or warm part of a meal. Sometimes I cook this at night so the rice can be ready in the morning for recipes like the Zippy Breakfast.

GADGETS are something you can get into, once you are committed to preparing mostly raw foods for your meals. Vegetables are beautiful and colorful, and presentation is always important to make the food look appetizing. I have a French mandolin for doing extra fancy cuts on veggies, and also a small hand machine that can make angel-hair pasta out of vegetables like squash. I also use a salad spinner to wash and dry greens before putting them into salads or wraps.

A FOOD DEHYDRATOR is a wonderful way to serve food warm, but not cooked, and also makes it easy to keep fresh dried veggies in your pantry. I use an Excalibur® brand and like how the air circulates throughout each tray, rather than just coming from the bottom up. The Excalibur® also comes with flexible, teflex liners that make it easy to lift off foods after they have dried. It is also a great way to warm up patés and loaf-type recipes before serving.

Although I don't use a small COFFEE GRINDER, they are great to grind smaller portions of nuts, seeds, and grains into fine powders. They are inexpensive and would make an excellent, economical grinder if you are preparing food for one or two people, or if you are traveling and doing your own cooking.

## Let's Go Shopping

Buying organically grown produce is the first priority because of its higher nutrient value, as much as 300 percent greater than non-organic. When organic is not available, get the freshest produce you can and wash the sprays off the food before you use it. You can find spray washes for vegetables in your local health food store, or you can soak them in water with chlorine dioxide ($ClO_2$) added, 20 drops to a gallon.

The following are items I keep in my pantry and fridge, so I have everything on hand when preparing delicious alkalizing meals.

# Ingredients

I love the spices and spice combinations put out by Spice Hunter, so these are mainly what I stock. Spice Hunter takes the guesswork out of how much to use in a dish by balancing the spices together and often giving a clue, by the name, as to when to use it, e.g. Mexican Seasoning. Here are some of my favorites:

**Spices (by Spice Hunter)**
The Zip (comes in mild, medium, and hot)
Spicy Garlic Bread Seasoning
Mexican Seasoning
Cowboy Barbecue Rub
California Pizza Seasoning
Pesto Seasoning
Deliciously Dill
Thai Seasoning
Italian Spice Blend
Jamaican Jerk Blend
Pasta Seasoning
Szechwan Seasoning
Vegetable Rub
Garam Masala
Curry Seasoning
Herbes De Provence
Tandoori Blend
All Purpose Blend

**Other Spices**
Real Salt™ (an alkalizing salt)
Bragg™ Liquid Aminos
Lemons and Limes (fresh)
Cumin
Cinnamon
Garlic (fresh cloves and granulated)
Ginger (fresh root is best; I keep one in the freezer and grate it for recipes)
Onion (fresh and flakes
Parsley (fresh and flakes)

**Seeds—always raw**
Flax
Sesame
Sunflower
Pumpkin
Sprouting combinations

**Nuts—always raw**
Almonds
Hazelnuts
Pecans
Pine Nuts

Brazil Nuts
Macadamia

**Grains**
Spelt
Buckwheat
Millet
Kamut
Quinoa
Amaranth

**Beans**
Adzuki
Lentils
Mung
Cranberry
Black
Black-eyed
Garbanzo
Pinto
Kidney

**Sea Vegetables**
Nori sheets
Dulse flakes
Aramie

**Fresh Vegetables**
Baby Greens
Larger Leafy Greens (romaine, red leaf, butter leaf, red oak, etc.)
Broccoli
Spinach
Kale
Red and Green Cabbage
Celery
Parsley
Carrots
Cucumber
Cauliflower
Squash
Zucchini
Sprouts (all kinds, sunflower are my favorite)
Beets
Radishes
Onions
Chili Peppers

**Fresh Fruits**
Avocado
Tomato
Lemon

Lime
Red, Green, Yellow, Orange Bell Peppers

**Other Items**
Rice Dream® Milk or Soy Milk
Almond Milk
Oils (Olive, Flax Seed, Udo's Choice® blend)
Vegetable Broth (I use Pacific Foods of Oregon brand)
Tahini (raw)
Hummus (I love Marantha brand)
Almond Butter (raw, Marantha brand)
Sun-dried Tomatoes, packed in olive oil
Flours (whole wheat, unbleached white, spelt, brown rice, millet, etc.)
Roasted Bell Peppers packed in oil
LaVosch crackers
Sprouted Wheat Tortillas (I use Alvarado St. brand)
Soba Noodles (found in your health food store)

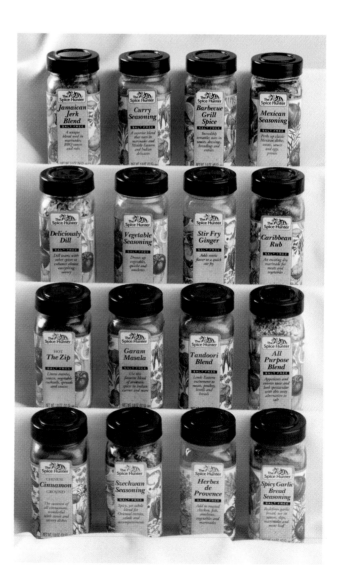

You don't need to go out and buy everything on this list at once. Get a few items from each category. Let it be an adventuresome journey to create a kitchen with alkalizing food choices for you and your loved ones!

# A Note on Healthy, Essential Fats

One of the most dangerous modern-day fad diets is the "No-fat" diet. People who don't realize the great role GOOD fats play in our bodies, open themselves up to degeneration and nutritional deficiencies by choosing never to eat fat. The body needs essential fatty acids (omega 3s and omega 6s) which are found in the highest concentration in flax seed oil, borage seed oil, hemp seed oil, Udo's Choice® and other combination oils found in your health food store.

As their name implies, essential fatty acids are vital to good health. They are the building-blocks of necessary fats and strengthen the cell wall, since cell walls have a biolipid (fat) layer. They strengthen immune cells, help lubricate joints, insulate the body against heat loss, provide energy, and are transformed by the body into hormone-like prostaglandins, necessary for energy metabolism and cardiovascular and immune system health. Prostaglandins have been shown through research to protect against heart disease, stroke, high blood pressure, arteriosclerosis, and blood clots.

Adding these good essential fats to your diet could also provide relief from arthritis, asthma, PMS, allergies, skin conditions, and improve brain function and some behavior disorders.

Nuts, seeds, and avocados are also good sources of healthy fats. The polyunsaturated fats support cell wall integrity and hormonal balance. The monounsaturated fats are used for energy purposes.

So, make like the Tin Man in the Wizard of Oz and "Oil up!"

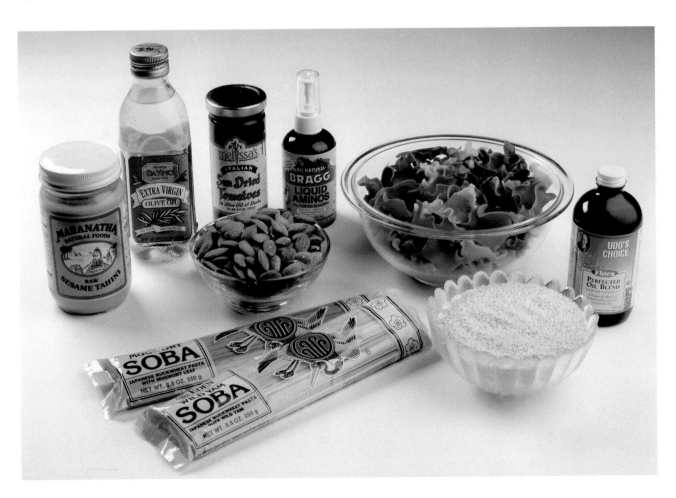

# Shelley's "Shortcuts"

Here are some tricks of the trade that make arranging alkalizing meals quick and easy:

1. Make a huge salad and keep it in the fridge for building the 70–80 percent foundational part of your meals. I make one that will last about three days and fill it with goodies like spinach, red onions, pine nuts, tofu cubes, shredded carrot and beet, radishes, and sunflower seed sprouts. This way I can grab a great salad or fill a wrap quickly. It's also good to have on hand when kids come home from school with that ravenous appetite.
2. Store a selection of your favorite spices in your pantry. I prefer the spice combinations that Spice Hunter offers. My favorite is "The Zip." Others I use frequently are Garlic Herb Bread Seasoning, Italian Pizza Seasoning, Lemon Pepper Blend, Cowboy Barbecue Rub, and Mexican Seasoning.
3. Keep a bowl of soaked almonds in the fridge. Cover with plenty of water, and change the water daily. They will keep for about five days. These are great, sweet, crunchy snacks, and also good for whipping up some nut milk in a hurry. I throw them on salads instead of croutons.
4. Mix up a batch of your favorite spread like pesto, Mock Mayo, hummus, or nut-spreads, and have on hand for quick dipping on veggie crackers, to top steamed veggies, or to spread on tortillas when making wraps. You can also find some good ones in your local health food store, but watch labels, and try to get dairyless pesto.
5. Make enough of your favorite salad dressings to last all week. Many of the spread recipes can be thinned with veggie juice or oil to be used as salad dressings also. Also, dressing recipes can be thickened with ground psyllium seed powder, agar agar, or kudzu root (found in your health food store).

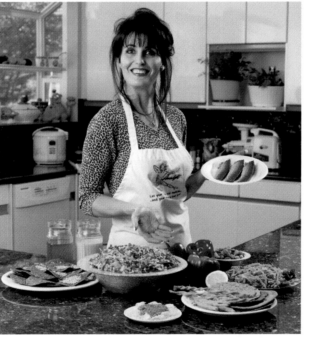

6. Double or triple some of the cooked recipes, like the Super Tortillas, Tofu Italian Mock Meatballs, or Baked Falafel Fritters, and freeze them. Then you have them on hand to complement your alkalizing meals, or to pop into your mouth for a quick on-the-run snack.
7. Keep lemons and limes on hand to use as a vinegar substitution and to squeeze into your drinking water all day long (highly alkalizing). I use lemons in almost every dish I serve.
8. Take a few packages of Sprouted Wheat Tortillas and set them out to dry or bake them in a low-heat oven. When crisp, but not browned, grind them in your food processor or blender until they are like flour. Then you have them ready to substitute when a recipe calls for bread crumbs or white flour. Store in an airtight container.
9. Keep the following items in the freezer for easy thaw access: raw nuts like almonds, hazelnuts, pecans, pine nuts; dried herbs like basil and oregano; also good oils like Udo's Choice® and flax seed oil. Fresh frozen ginger can be grated on a hand grater for a recipe, then put back in the freezer. This is a great way to have fresh lemon ginger tea after a nice meal.
10. Keep a rice cooker on the counter with a fresh batch of steamed legumes or grains such as rice, buckwheat groats, millet, or spelt to complement your meal with the 20–30 percent grounding, warm part of your meal.
11. Stock your fridge or pantry with good water, like distilled or reverse osmosis water, and superhydrate, especially in between meals. When eating 80 percent alkalizing meals, you may not feel a need to drink with meals, as raw alkalizing vegetables are between 70–90 percent high water content.
12. Learn to do your own sprouting and keep fresh sprouts on hand. They can be a great snack or nutritional booster to any meal.

# Metric Conversion Chart

| IMPERIAL | METRIC |
|---|---|
| 1 inch | 2.54 centimeters |
| 1 ounce | 28.35 grams |
| 1 pound | 0.45 kilogram |
| 1/2 teaspoon | 1.25 milliliters |
| 1/2 teaspoon | 2.5 milliliters |
| 1 teaspoon | 5 milliliters |
| 1 tablespoon | 15 milliliters |
| 1/3 cup | 80 milliliters |
| 1/2 cup | 120 milliliters |
| 1 cup | 250 milliliters |
| 1 pint   (2 cups) | 480 milliliters |
| 1 quart (4 cups; 32 ounces) | 960 milliliters |
| 1 gallon (4 quarts) | 3.84 liters |
| 16 fluid ounces | 0.47 liter |
| 32° Fahrenheit | 0* Celsius |

Note: Conversions in this book from imperial to metric are not exact. They have been rounded to the nearest standard measure for convenience. To prepare recipes more exactly, follow the imperial measures.

# Resources

Spice Hunter Spices
San Luis Obispo, CA 93401
800-444-3061
www.spicehunter.com

Vita Mix Blenders
8615 Usher Road
Cleveland, Ohio 44138-2199
800 848-2649
www.vita-mix.com

Green Power Juicers
Orders: 888-254-7336
Inquiries: 562-940-4241
Fax: 562-940-4240
www.greenpower.com

Organic Food-Mail Order
Diamond Organics
P.O. Box 2159
Freedom, CA 95019
Shop toll-free: 888-674-2642
Shop by Fax: 888-888-6777
Organics@diamondorganics.com

Life Sprouts
P.O. Box 150
Paradise, Utah 94321
435-245-3891
www.lifesprouts.net

Cutco  Knives
www.cutco.com

The Robert O. Young
Research Center
134 E. 200 No.
Alpine, Utah  84004
801-756-7850
Orders: 800-677-0997
*A clearing house of information for many products used in the House of Health Recipe Book and services*

Real Salt@
Redmond Minerals, Inc.
800-367-7258
www.realsalt.com

# Vegetable Juices and Nut Milks

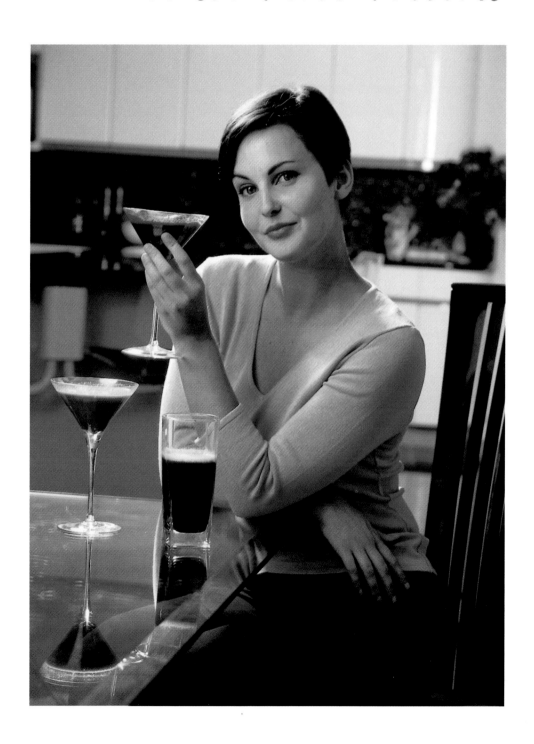

Fresh vegetable juicing is a wonderful concentrated way to alkalize! When drinking raw, alkalizing vegetable juices, the body can assimilate the nutrients most rapidly. When the juice is mostly made up of green vegetables, the alkalizing effects are optimal. The preference would be to use organic vegetables whenever possible. Green leafy and other green vegetables have the highest amounts of chlorophyll, making them molecularly structured most like our own hemoglobin (blood). If you are not accustomed to mostly green juice, then add some carrot or beet (which are higher in sugar) moderately, until your tastebuds become more accustomed to the subtler sweet taste of green juices. Red, yellow, or orange bell peppers also add a hint of sweetness.

Foods that can be juiced nicely are: all green vegetables (e.g., celery, lettuce, cucumber, broccoli, cabbage, zucchini, green beans), beet greens, bell peppers, sprouts, jicama, garlic, ginger, radish, tomatoes. Carrot, beet, butternut squash, and sweet potatoes can be used in moderation. There are many different juicers at all prices on the market, some requiring less clean-up than others. To juice grasses or parsley, a high-powered juicer is required, e.g., the Green Power® Juice Extractor, which is unique in that it also ionizes the juice.

# Juicing Recipes

## Vegetable Juice

Greens such as Wheat Grass, Celery, Kale, Lettuce, Spinach, Parsley, Bell Peppers, Cabbage, Cucumber, and Sprouts of any kind, etc.
(A little raw ginger, garlic, or flax seed oil can be added to taste.)

## Vegetable/Grass Drink

1–3 oz. Carrot Juice (3 carrots-or less, try to keep at least 80% green)
3 oz. Celery Juice (2 large stalks)
1/2 oz. Parsley Juice (5 sprigs)
1 1/2 oz. Wheat Grass Juice

## Wheat-Beet Juice

1 1/2 oz. Wheat Grass Juice
1 oz. Beet Juice
6 oz. Cucumber Juice

## Potassium Special

3 oz. Carrot
4 oz. Celery
2 oz. Parsley
3 oz. Spinach

## Insulin Generator

3 oz. Brussels Sprouts
3–6 oz. Carrot
3 oz. String Bean
4 oz. Lettuce

## Skin Cleanse

4 oz. Potato
4 oz. Celery
3–6 oz. Carrot
2 oz. Watercress

## Blood Builder

8 oz. Celery
3 oz. Cucumber
2 oz. Parsley
3 oz. Spinach

## High Vitamin C & E Drink

6 oz. Spinach
2 oz. Lettuce
2 oz. Watercress
4 oz. Carrots
2 oz. Green Peppers

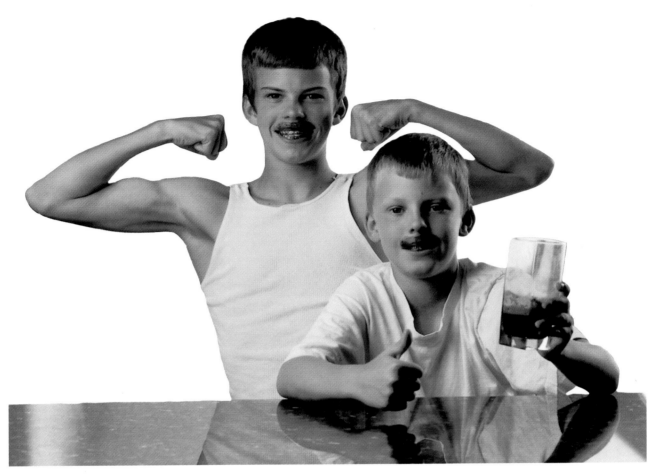

# *Greens—They Do the Body Good!*

## Green Power Cocktail

4 cups Sprouts
4 cups Green Tops
1 cup Kale
1 cup Beets
1/2 cup Wheat Grass

## Basic Green Drink

4 cups Alfalfa and/or other Sprouts
4 cups Sunflower and Buckwheat Greens
1/2 cup Carrots
1/2 cup sweet Red Peppers
1/4 cup Parsley
1 cup Cucumber
Add 1 bunch Wheat Grass (about 3/4" thick), if desired

## Spring Green Drink

4 cups Sprouts
4 cups Greens
1/2 cup Dandelion Greens
1/4 cup Scallion
1 cup Carrots

## Garden Green Drink

4 cups Sprouts
4 cups Green Tops
2 cups Kale or Collard Greens
1 cup Celery

# Nut & Seed Milks

When phasing off from dairy foods, nut milks or sesame milk are a wonderful way to keep a creamy texture in your dressings and soups, or just to drink for a snack. Their richness and sweetness can be varied, depending on how you dilute them to taste. They are also good sources of protein and calcium. I mostly use almond, sesame, and occasionally coconut milk. If you don't want to make your own, Pacific Foods of Oregon puts out a nice almond milk in a carton.

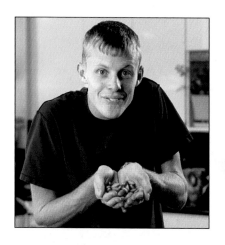

*Almonds—Delicious and Fun!*

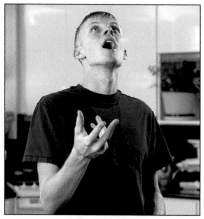

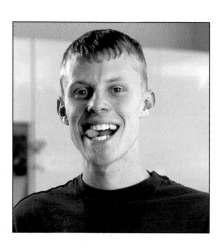

## Almond Milk

**1/2 cup Almonds (soaked 12 hours)**
**1/2 cup Pine Nuts (soaked 6 hours)**
**1 cup spring or filtered Water**

Soak almonds and pine nuts for 12 hours. Put in blender and pulverize. Add one cup of water gradually, while continuing to blend on high. Strain through a fine strainer or cheesecloth (you can use the almond pulp as a body scrub). This milk will keep for three to four days. It is great on hot grains such as quinoa, buckwheat groats, millet, or amaranth. We like to add some soaked almonds to our grains for "crunch." You can thin further with more water if desired.

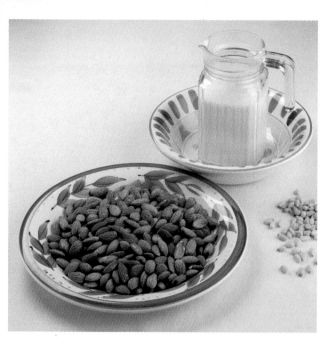

## Quick Tahini Milk

**2–4 Tbs. Tahini (raw)**
**1 cup Water**

Tahini is a butter made from hulled sesame seeds, usually used as a spread. It also makes a very nutritious milk which is high in calcium and protein. In a blender, combine 2 Tbs. of tahini with water. Blend thoroughly and taste. Add additional tahini and blend again for a richer milk. This milk will keep for three to four days.

# Breakfast Must Change!

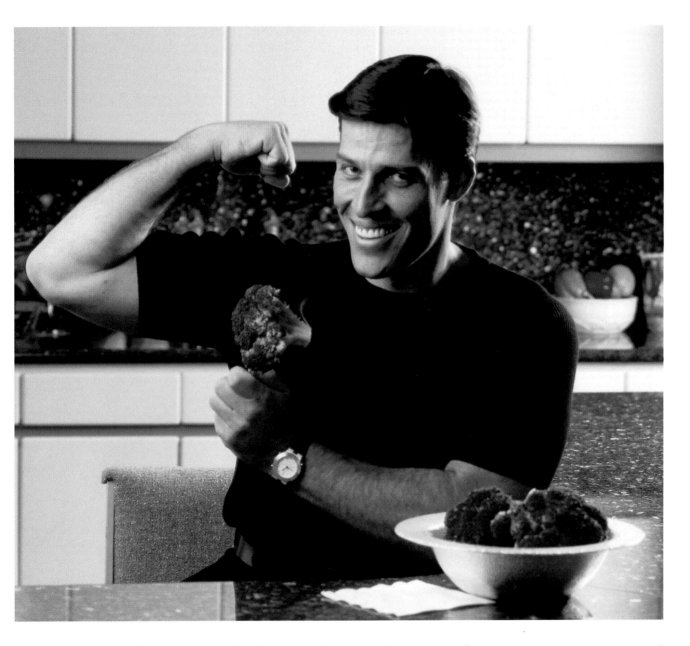

## *Breakfast of a Champion!*

*One personal choice seems to influence long-term health prospects more than any other—WHAT WE EAT.*

**—C. Everett Koop, M.D.**
Surgeon General

As mentioned in the Introduction, most of the conventional choices for breakfast meals are acid-forming. Here are some alkalizing menus that make a great way to start off your day. I know it may seem strange at first to consider a salad or soup for breakfast, but just try it for a couple of weeks. If you're like most people, you may find that an alkalizing breakfast provides a great amount of energy and burns longer into the mid-day without the drop in blood sugar that so commonly occurs with a starchy, sugary breakfast. My personal favorite is the "Zippy Breakfast" recipe. Everyone I've ever served this to has loved it! The combo of the avocado/ tomato/lemon-lime, and my favorite spice, "The Zip," makes it a real eye-opener. I usually don't feel hungry until 2:00 or 3:00 in the afternoon after having this great breakfast. In the summer months, when it's hotter, a nice salad with lots of sprouts or a green drink is our breakfast. In the winter, vegetable soup is a nice warm alkalizing breakfast. Remember, this will take some transition time, and some old traditions will have to be changed. While traveling in Israel, I was so pleased to see salads, tabouli, soups, and many alkalizing dishes laid out in their breakfast buffets. Also, please remember that any of these breakfast recipes make a great alkalizing snack, lunch, or dinner too!

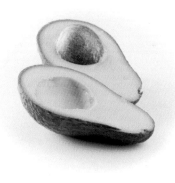

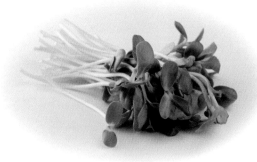

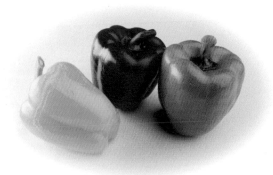

# AsparaZincado Soup

*15 minutes to prepare. Serves 3–5. This great soup is rich in zinc and has a rich tomatoeeee flavor!*

12 stalks medium Asparagus (or 17 thin stalks)

1 Avocado

5–6 large Tomatoes

1 cup fresh Parsley

3–5 Sun-dried Tomatoes (bottled in olive oil)

1/4 cup dried Onion

4 cloves fresh Garlic

1 Red Bell Pepper

Bragg™ Liquid Aminos to taste

1–2 tsp. Spice Hunter's Herbes de Provence

2 tsp. Spice Hunter's Deliciously Dill

2 Lemons or Limes, cut in thin slices

Trim and dice the tips from the asparagus and set aside for a garnish. In a food processor or Vita-Mix® blend the asparagus and red tomatoes, parsley, dried tomatoes, spices, garlic, onion, and red bell pepper. Then blend in the avocado until soup is smooth and creamy. Warm in an electric skillet and garnish with lemon or lime slices on top. Season with Bragg's to taste or serve cold in the summertime. Sprinkle diced asparagus tips on top just before serving. Yummy!

# Casserole de Cauliflower

*20 minutes to prepare. Serves 4–6. This dish is a lot like couscous in texture and makes a great breakfast, lunch, or dinner side dish.*

1. In an electric skillet or fry pan, warm the oil, cumin, and turmeric.

2. Keeping the temperature on warm or low, add the onion and allow the flavors to blend for 2–4 minutes, then add the water and warm.

3. In a food processor fitted with an S-blade, process the cauliflower into very small pieces (like couscous). Also process the sun-dried tomatoes into fine, small pieces.

4. Add the cauliflower to the skillet and gradually warm, adding the parsley, bell pepper, garlic, sun-dried tomatoes and pine nuts. Season with Bragg™ Aminos to taste. Enjoy!

2 tsp. Oil (Olive, Flax Seed, or Udo's Choice®)

2–4 tsp. Cumin

1–2 tsp. Turmeric

1/2 Yellow or Red Onion, finely minced

1 cup Water

Flowerets from 1 very large or 2 small Cauliflowers

4 Tbs. fresh Parsley, minced

1/2 cup raw Pine Nuts

7–8 Sun-dried Tomatoes (Melissa's brand are packed in olive oil)

Bragg™ Liquid Aminos to taste

Lemon or Lime Juice to taste

2 cloves Garlic, minced

1 Red Bell Pepper, chopped

# Creamy or Crunchy Broccoli Soup

*15 minutes to prepare. Serves 4–6. This high-protein soup is for broccoli lovers!*

**2 cups Vegetable Stock or Water**
**3–4 cups Broccoli, chopped**
**1 Red Bell Pepper, chopped**
**2 Red or Yellow Onions, chopped**
**1 Avocado**
**1–2 stalks of Celery, cut in large pieces**
**Bragg™ Liquid Aminos to taste**
**Cumin and Ginger to taste (experiment with different spices!)**

1. In an electric skillet, warm 2 cups of water or stock, keeping the temperature at or below 118° (finger test). Add the chopped broccoli and warm for 5 minutes.

2. In a blender, purée the warmed broccoli, bell pepper, onion, avocado, and celery, thinning with additional water if necessary to achieve the desired consistency. If desired, save the broccoli stalks, peeling off the tough outer skin; process them in a food processor until they are small chunks, and add to the soup just before serving to add crunch!

3. Serve warm, flavoring with Bragg's, fresh ginger, cumin, or any other spices you like. Add a slice of lemon on top to garnish.

# Zippy Breakfast (our favorite!)

*Serves 1.*

**1–2 Cups Cooked Rice or Grain of your choice (I use basmati, brown, or wild rice, or buckwheat)**
**Juice of 1 Lemon or Lime (or both)**
**1–2 tsp. Oil (Flax, Udo's, Olive)**
**1–2 tsp. Bragg™ Liquid Aminos**
**1 Avocado, sliced**
**1 firm Tomato**
**The Zip (Spice Hunter) to taste**

Start with the warm rice in a bowl. Slice the avocado and tomato on top. Then drizzle the oil, Bragg™ Aminos, and lemon juice over the top. Sprinkle with "Zip" to taste. For other grain choices, try buckwheat groats, millet, quinoa, or spelt.

Variation: Sometimes I throw in some chopped red bell pepper, sunflower seed sprouts, and soaked almonds over the top for extra crunch! Enjoy!

# Zippy Breakfast

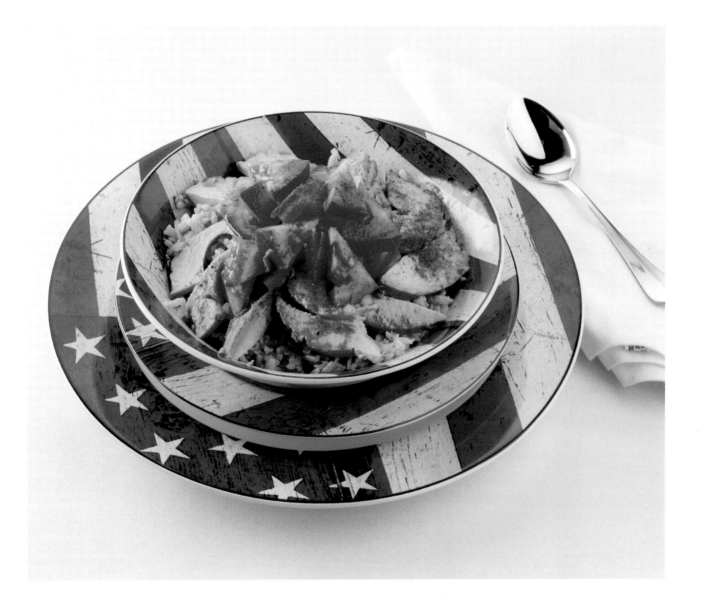

# Popeye Soup

*10 minutes to prepare. Serves 4–6. This is a wonderful alkalizing soup because of the cucumbers and greens. Serve warm with a fresh tortilla for dipping.*

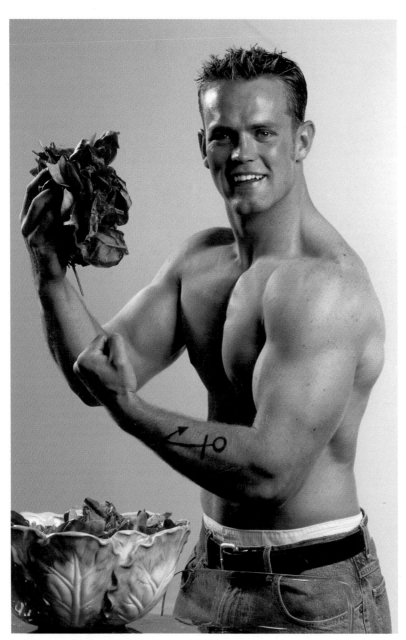

**"I'm strong to the finish 'cause I eats raw spinach."**

1 Avocado

1 cup Water or Vegetable Stock (Pacific Foods of Oregon brand is yeast free)

2 Cucumbers, unwaxed

1 cup fresh raw Spinach

2 Green Onions

1 clove Garlic

1/3 Red Bell Pepper

Bragg™ Liquid Aminos or Real Salt™ to taste

Mid-Eastern Spices (Spice Hunter's Garam Masala, 1/2–1 tsp., Curry Seasoning, 1/2–1 tsp., and "Zip," 1/2 tsp.)

Fresh Lime Juice to taste

(4 spearmint leaves to garnish)

1. In a Vita-Mix® or blender, add the avocado and half of the water or stock, and purée, then add the rest of the ingredients (except the spearmint leaves) one at a time, blending to desired thickness and thinning with the remaining water if desired. Add Bragg™ Aminos or Real Salt™ to taste, and flavor with spices and lime juice to your desire. You might add a couple of minced sun-dried tomatoes too. Experiment! Also this soup is good while on the cleanse phase of Dr. Young's Complete Program and Diet™.

2. Warming options: This soup can be served warm or cold. If blending in a Vita-Mix®, the longer you blend, the warmer the soup will get. If you do not have a Vita-Mix®, you can carefully warm the soup (not cook it) in an electric or stove-top skillet on low heat. Only warm the soup until you can hold your finger in it without having to pull it out. This will keep the food at about 118° which will keep the food raw, but warm. Serve with mint leaves on top. Enjoy!

# CHAPTER 4

# *Foundation*

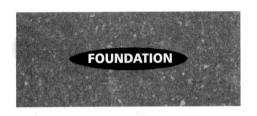

FOUNDATION

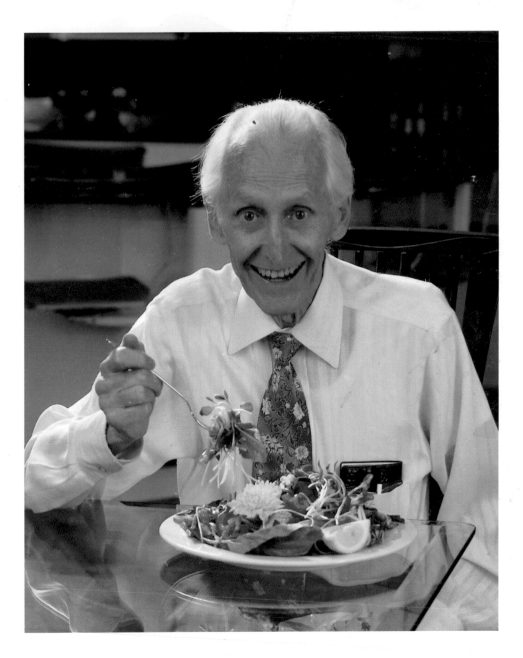

*The closer food is to the natural sun energy, the higher it is in all levels of nutritional value for the human organism.*

—Dr. Klinik Bircher-Benner

## Salad, Soup, and Raw Food Recipes

For the most part, the following recipes would be considered 90–100 percent alkalizing and should be used for the 70–80 percent alkalizing part of your meal arrangement. These recipes would also be the ones to stay on during a cleanse or when dealing with a serious state of health imbalance or symptomatology. Again, the live raw foods contained in these recipes, and the fresh juicing recipes, will provide the best energy-giving substances and support to the bloodstream. When you build your personal House of Health, think of these recipes as the FOUNDATION of your House—the STRONGEST and most supportive part of you!

Traditionally a salad has been used as a "token" to the side of the main dish or as an appetizer before a heavier main course. To continually maintain an alkaline blood pH, the thinking needs to change to regard these wonderful, beautiful salads as the MAIN COURSE. Other vegan dishes, including grains, soups, tortillas, patés, and other warmed and cooked foods, should complement and be the side dish to the salad. Some people think making a great salad involves a lot of work, and true, it may take more time than a "zapped" microwave meal; however, the nutritional and alkalizing effects will be well worth the small amount of extra time you invest in yourself and your loved ones. Just remember YOU ARE WORTH IT! Also, a big salad, once made and stored airtight in the fridge, will last for about three days and still be fresh. Just be sure to wash and spin-dry your greens so they will stay crisp.

Get creative with salads too! You can make them extra hearty by adding tofu cubes, pine nuts, soaked almonds, sprouts, or dehydrated grains like the Crispy Buckwheat Groats. I've even cut up some baked warm falafel and added this to my salad in place of croutons! Also, to satisfy the need for crunch, serve the veggie crackers or baked tortillas. Spread some hummus on a sprouted wheat tortilla and roll it up to the side of your salad for a more filling meal.

Salads are my favorite meal, and very often I'll have one for breakfast!

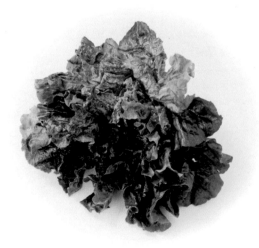

# Creamy or Crunchy Broccoli Soup

*15 minutes to prepare. Serves 4–6. This high-protein soup is for broccoli lovers!*

1. In an electric skillet, warm 2 cups of water or stock, keeping the temperature at or below 118° (finger test). Add the chopped broccoli and warm for 5 minutes.

2. In a blender, purée the warmed broccoli, bell pepper, onion, avocado, and celery, thinning with additional water if necessary to achieve the desired consistency. If desired, save the broccoli stalks, peeling off the tough outer skin; process them in a food processor until they are small chunks, and add to the soup just before serving to add crunch!

3. Serve warm, flavoring with Bragg's, fresh ginger, cumin, or any other spices you like. Add a slice of lemon on top to garnish.

**2 cups Vegetable Stock or Water**
**3–4 cups Broccoli, chopped**
**1 Red Bell Pepper, chopped**
**2 Red or Yellow Onions, chopped**
**1 Avocado**
**1–2 stalks of Celery, cut in large pieces**
**Bragg™ Liquid Aminos or Real Salt™ to taste**
**Cumin and Ginger to taste (experiment with different spices!)**

# Gazpacho

*Yields six 3/4-cup servings.*

Combine all ingredients. Cover and chill overnight.

**4 cups fresh Tomato Juice (you make)**
**1/2 cup Cucumber, chopped**
**1/4 cup Green Bell Pepper, chopped**
**1/4 cup Celery, finely chopped**
**1 Tbs. Olive Oil**
**1/2 tsp. Pepper**
**1 tsp. Basil**
**1/2 tsp. Garlic, minced**

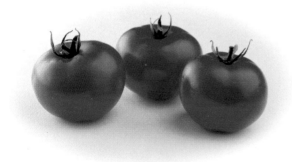

# Anti-Cancer Soup

*20 minutes to prepare. Serves 2.*

Soak caraway seeds in pure water 24 hours prior to use, then pour off liquid. Put finely cut broccoli flowers and thinly sliced, peeled stems in sauce pan with cover. Grate cabbage and carrots over broccoli, and add caraway. Blend onions in 2 cups hot water, and pour broth over veggies. Cover, let steam 5 minutes, garnishing with dill and sliced red pepper.

**2 cups hot Water**
**2 Green Onions, cut**
**2 Tbs. Caraway Seed**
**2 Carrots**
**2 slices each, Purple and Green Cabbage**
**2 Broccoli Stalks**
**1 Red Pepper, sliced**
**3 Tbs. fresh Dill Weed**

# Green Raw Soup

*This is wonderfully alkalizing soup that I prefer served cold in the summer months and warmed in the winter months. It's energizing and easy to digest.*

1–2 Avocados

1–2 Cucumbers, peeled and seeded

1 Jalapeño Pepper, seeded

1/2 Yellow Onion, diced

Juice of 1/2 Lemon

1–2 cups light Vegetable Stock or Water

3 cloves roasted Garlic

1 Tbs. fresh Cilantro

1 Tbs. fresh Parsley

1 Carrot, finely diced

Purée all ingredients (except onions and carrots) in a food processor or Vita-Mix®. Add more or less water to desired consistency. Add onions and raw crunch carrot bits at the end for a garnish. Yum!

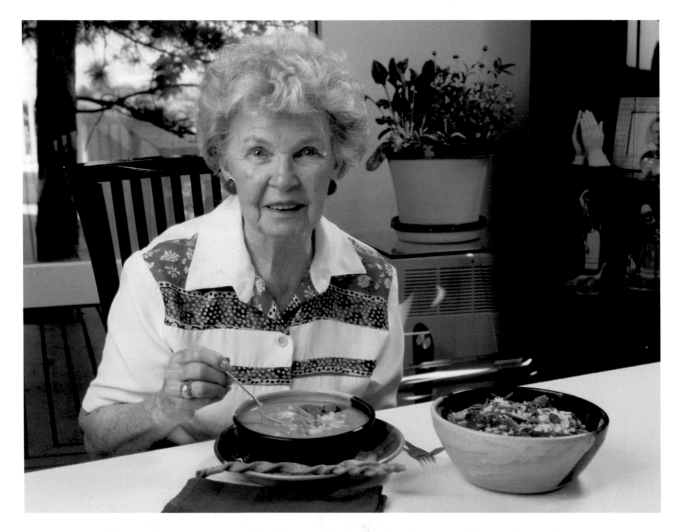

*Served warm or cold, Green Raw Soup is one of our favorites!*

# AsparaZincado Soup

*15 minutes to prepare. Serves 3–5. This great soup is rich in zinc and has a rich tomatoeeee flavor!*

Trim and dice the tips from the asparagus and set aside for a garnish. In a food processor or Vita-Mix® blend the asparagus and red tomatoes, parsley, dried tomatoes, spices, garlic, onion, and red bell pepper. Then blend in the avocado until soup is smooth and creamy. Warm in an electric skillet and garnish with lemon or lime slices on top. Season with Bragg's to taste or serve cold in the summertime. Sprinkle diced asparagus tips on top of soup just before serving. Yummy!

12 stalks medium Asparagus (or 17 thin stalks)
1 Avocado
5–6 large Tomatoes
1 cup fresh Parsley
3–5 Sun-dried Tomatoes (bottled in olive oil)
1/4 cup dried Onion
4 cloves fresh Garlic
1 Red Bell Pepper
Bragg™ Liquid Aminos to taste
1–2 tsp. Spice Hunter's Herbes de Provence
2 tsp. Spice Hunter's Deliciously Dill
2 Lemons or Limes, cut in thin slices

*AsparaZincado Soup*

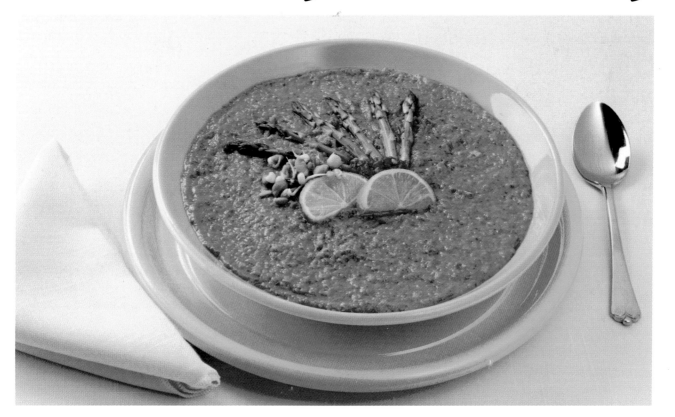

# All-Vegetable Cocktail

1 pt. fresh Tomatoes
1/2 tsp. Garlic
1 Cucumber, sliced
1 Green Pepper
Sprigs of fresh Parsley
1/4 Onion, sliced
2–3 Lettuce Leaves
1/2 tsp. Ginger

Blend all ingredients in a blender on low speed.

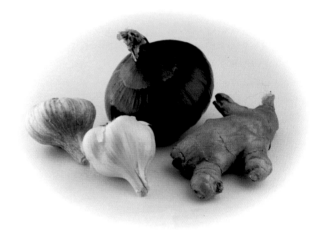

# Vegetable Minestrone Soup

1 small Cabbage
1 Red Bell Pepper
1 Onion
2 Carrots
2 Celery
1 Zucchini
1 Yellow Summer Squash

Cut vegetables as preferred. Cover carrots and celery with water in soup pot. Cook gently until they just begin to "give," then add remaining ingredients. Do not overcook.

Serve hot with flax seed oil, Bragg™ Liquid Aminos, and cayenne pepper to taste.

# Chunky Veggie Soup

*Serves 4.*

2 1/2 cups fresh Carrot Juice
1 Avocado
6–8 Celery Stalks
2 Carrots
1 Summer Squash
Small bunch of Arugala
Spice options: Parsley, Basil, Coriander

For broth, blend carrot juice, avocado, and 3–4 celery stalks. Grate squash and carrots and celery, adding finely chopped arugala and other fresh green spices last. Serve in a bowl or cup; decorate with fresh herbs.

# Healing Soup

*This soup is especially soothing when tired, stressed, or sick with cold or flu, and is very anti-fungal.*

Chop and crush garlic cloves into small diced pieces and lightly steam-fry. Set aside. Put whole onion in water in a deep pan, simmer until onion is transparent (approx. 1 hour). Add garlic and yeast-free instant vegetable broth. Slice cucumber (and optional veggies) and add
to soup. Simmer 10–15 minutes. Add fresh ginger, cilantro, and Real Salt™ to taste.

Variation: You could also bring the water to a boil, then take it off the burner and drop assorted finely chopped veggies into the water. This would just warm, but not cook the vegetables.

2–3 whole Garlic cloves
1 large Onion
3 Tbs. yeast-free instant Vegetable Broth
2–3 quarts Water or Veggie Broth (Pacific Brand)
1 Cucumber (optional: Carrots, Cabbage, Celery, and any other veggies desired)
2 Tbs. fresh Cilantro
2 tsp. fresh grated Ginger
Real Salt™ to taste

# Celery Soup

Cook celery until tenderized. Add water and broth mix. Pour all into blender. Blend 15–20 seconds. Reheat and serve. Use flax seed oil, Bragg™ Liquid Aminos, and cayenne pepper, to taste.

4–5 stalks Celery (including leaves, if fresh)
3 cups pure Water
2 Tbs. yeast-free instant Vegetable Broth

# Special Carrot Soup

*Serves 4.*

1. In a saucepan, steam-fry the onion. Add carrots, garlic, mustard seeds, spices, and salt. Cook for 2 to 3 minutes, stirring constantly. Add 1/2 cup water, cover, and simmer until carrots begin to soften. Let cool.

2. In a large saucepan bring 5 cups water to a near boil and reduce to medium. Stir kuzu root into 1 cup cool water. Slowly pour into heated water and cook until thick.

3. Place cooled carrot mixture in a blender and purée on low speed until smooth, adding a bit of water if needed. Add purée to thickened water and cook for 5 minutes, stirring as needed. Add lecithin, and stir for a minute. Adjust thickness if desired.

4 large Carrots, sliced
1 small Onion, chopped
1 clove Garlic, minced
1/4 tsp. Turmeric, 1/4 tsp. Cumin
1/4 tsp. Ginger, 1/4 tsp. Mustard Seeds
1/4 tsp. Real Salt™
Pinch of ground Cinnamon
Pinch of Cayenne Pepper
7 cups Water
1/3 cup Kuzu root
1 tsp. Lecithin (liquid or powder)

# Popeye Soup

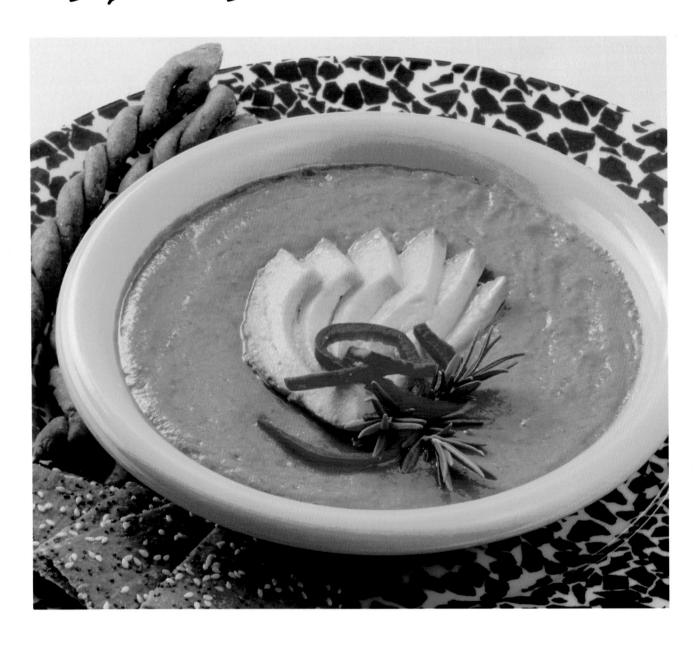

# Popeye Soup

*10 minutes to prepare. Serves 4–6. This is a wonderful alkalizing soup because of the cucumbers and greens. Serve warm with a fresh tortilla for dipping.*

1. In a Vita-Mix® or blender, add the avocado and half of the water or stock and purée, then add the rest of the ingredients (except the spearmint leaves) one at a time, blending to desired thickness and thinning with the remaining water if desired. Add Bragg™ Aminos or Real Salt ™ to taste, and flavor with spices and lime juice to your desire. You might add a couple of minced sun-dried tomatoes too. Experiment! Also this soup is good while on the InnerLight liquid cleanse.

2. Warming options: This soup can be served warm or cold. If blending in a Vita-Mix®, the longer you blend, the warmer the soup will get. If you do not have a Vita-Mix®, you can carefully warm the soup (not cook it) in an electric or stove-top skillet on low heat. Only warm the soup until you can hold your finger in it without having to pull it out. This will keep the food at about 118°, which will keep the food raw, but warm and not cooked. Serve with mint leaves on top. Enjoy!

1 Avocado

1 cup Water or Vegetable Stock (Pacific Foods of Oregon brand is yeast free)

2 Cucumbers, unwaxed

1 cup fresh raw Spinach

2 Green Onions

1 clove Garlic

1/3 Red Bell Pepper

Bragg™ Liquid Aminos or Real Salt™ to taste

Mid-Eastern Spices (Spice Hunter's Garam Masala, 1/2–1 tsp., Curry Seasoning, 1/2–1 tsp., and "Zip," 1/2 tsp.)

Fresh Lime Juice to taste

(4 spearmint leaves to garnish)

# Mock Split-Pea Soup

*Serves 4.*

Chop all vegetable ingredients in food processer and add to 4 cups of water or vegetable stock in a soup pot. Lighly simmer until vegetables are just softened—about 8–10 minutes—then put contents into a blender and thoroughly purée until thick, creamy texture is achieved. Add salt and seasonings. Serve warm.
Optional seasoning suggestions include 1/2 tsp. cumin, 1/2 tsp. dill, 1/2 tsp. herbs de provence, and a squirt or two of Bragg™.

2 Carrots, shaved

2 Celery Stalks, cut as desired

6 sprigs Parsley

1 Onion, chopped

4 cups Water

2 cups crisp-steamed Green Beans

1 1/2 cups crisp-steamed Asparagus

Dash of Mace

1 Bay Leaf

1 tsp. Vegetized or Real Salt™

# Zucchini Toss

Dressing:
1/4 cup Flax Seed Oil
2 Tbs. Real Salt™
Garlic clove(s) to taste, crushed
1/4 tsp. dried Tarragon Leaves

1 med. Red-Leaf Lettuce

1 small Romaine Lettuce

2 med. Zucchini, thinly sliced

1 cup Radishes, sliced

3 Green Onions, sliced

# Colorful Cabbage

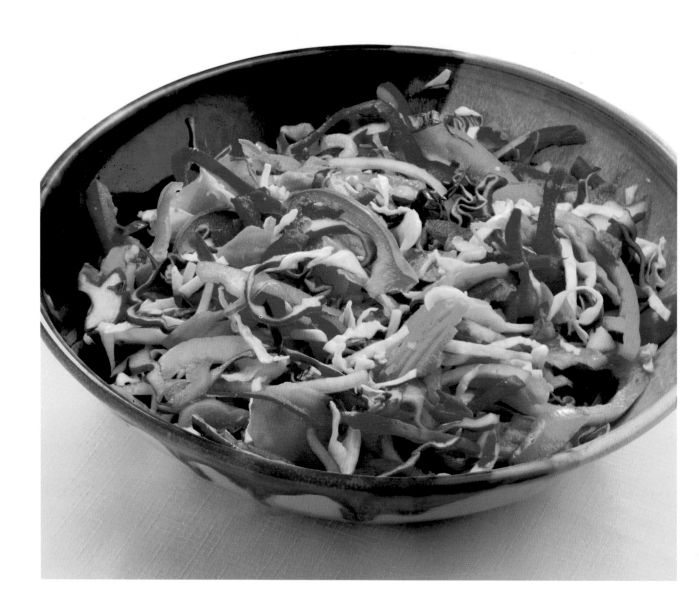

# Colorful Cabbage

*Serves 4. Cabbage is considered one of the most powerful therapeutic foods in the world. Many studies have linked eating cabbage with a reduction of cancer, especially colon cancer. Also, cabbage juice has been proven to help heal stomach ulcers, and prevent stomach cancer.*

In a bowl, combine the red and green cabbages, carrot, peppers, scallions, parsley, lemon juice, water, oil, dried pepper and Bragg™ Aminos. Toss thoroughly and let the flavors mix for at least a half-hour before serving.

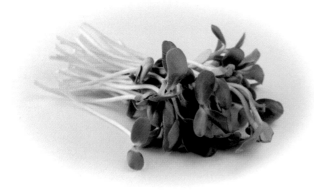

2 cups Red Cabbage, thinly sliced

2 cups Green Cabbage, thinly sliced

1 Carrot, grated

1 Red Pepper, slivered

1 Yellow Pepper, slivered

1 Green Pepper, slivered

1 Orange Pepper, slivered

4 Tbs. Scallions, chopped

4 Tbs. Parsley, minced

1/4 cup Lemon Juice

3 Tbs. water

1 Tbs. Oil (Extra Virgin Olive, Flax Seed, or Udo's Choice®)

1–2 tsp. dried Red Chili Pepper

Dash of Bragg™ Liquid Aminos

# Spring's Pesto

Combine all ingredients in a food processor (with an S-blade) or in a blender. Blend until smooth.

6 cloves Garlic

4 cups fresh Basil or 1 cup dried Basil

1 cup fresh Parsley

6 Tbs. raw Nuts (pine, almond, hazelnut, pumpkin) I use a combination and soak them overnight.

1 cup or more of Olive Oil

1/2 tsp. each of Real Salt™ and Pepper

2 Tbs. sun dried Tomatoes

# Spinach Salad

In a large bowl, combine the spinach, shallots, basil, red peppers, celery, cauliflower, radishes and pine nuts. Toss well. Top with Essential Dressing (see page 74).

1 head Spinach

1/2 cup Cauliflower, cut in small pieces

2 stalks Celery, chopped

6 Radishes, chopped

2 Shallots, chopped (or 1 small Red Onion)

1/2 cup chopped Basil

2 Red Peppers, chopped

4 Tbs. Pine Nuts

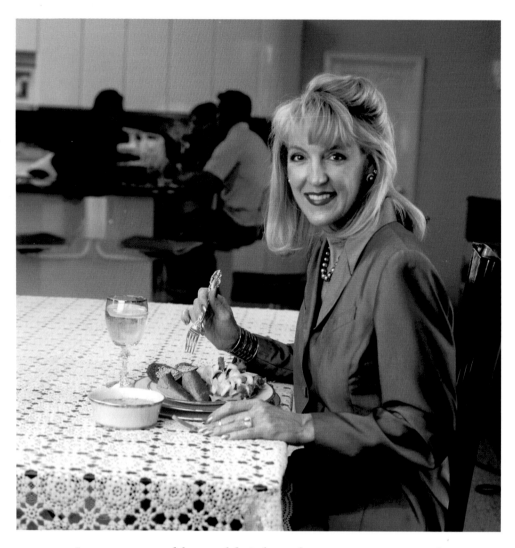

*Its raw vegetables and bright color arrangement make
Pretty Ribbon Quiche a favorite of all who try it!*

# Broccoli Salad

**1 head Broccoli**
**1 cup diced Celery**
**4 chopped Scallions**
**1 large Red Onion, chopped**
**1/3 cup Parsley Dressing or Flax Oil Dressing**

Cut raw broccoli into bite-size pieces. Mix all ingredients, chill one hour.

# *Pretty Ribbon Quiche*

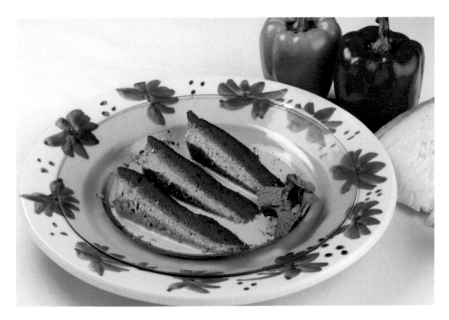

## Pretty Ribbon Quiche

*This recipe is beautiful with rich colors of raw veggies. It is set up by using psyllium seed powder. Use the Almond crust recipe from the Popeye Mousse Pie and build the three layers of the Ribbon Quiche in it.*

1. Put all ingredients in food processor except psyllium seed powder. Process until well blended and somewhat smooth. With the machine still running add the psyllium seed powder slowly. Mix well and pour this into the almond crust. Place in fridge to set up while you make layer 2.

2. Process carrots and orange bell pepper until smooth. With machine still running add psyllium seed powder and continue to process until well blended. Spread evenly over layer one and place back in fridge while you make layer 3.

3. Follow same directions as layer one and two and spread onto layer two. Place in fridge to finish chilling 4- 6 hours or overnight. Cut and serve with favorite garnish or dressing on top if desired. Ginger Almond dressing is nice.

**LAYER ONE**
2 1/2 cups Coarsely Chopped Spinach
2 1/2 cups Coarsely Chopped Green Cabbage
1/2 cup Fresh Lemon Juice
1/2 tsp. Real Salt™
1/2 cup Tofu (Firm)
1 Tbs. Red Onion, finely chopped
1 Tbs. Deliciously Dill (Spice Hunter)
1/2 cup Raw Pinenuts
1 1/2 tsp. Psyllium Seed Powder

**LAYER TWO**
1/3 cup Tofu (firm)
4–5 Carrots, chopped
1 Orange Bell Pepper
1/2–1 tsp. Psyllium Seed Powder

**LAYER THREE**
1/3 cup Tofu (firm)
2–3 medium Beets, peeled and chopped
1 Red Bell Pepper
1 small Tomato
1/2–1 tsp. Psyllium Seed Powder

# Rich Raw Tomato Sauce

*This is a wonderfully fresh tasting raw tomato sauce that goes great over pasta. I use it over raw Yellow crook neck Squash angel hair, which I make with a gadget called the Saladacco. It also is a wonderful dipping sauce too, and can be served cold or warmed but not cooked.*

**3–5 Sun Dried Tomatoes (I use Melissa's brand packed in Olive Oil)**

**4 fresh, firm Tomatoes, chopped**

**1/2 cup Fresh Basil, chopped**

**1 tsp. Dried Onion**

**1 tsp. Roasted Garlic**

**1 tsp. Real Salt™**

Put all ingredients in food processor and blend to desired consistency. Store in airtight container in refrigerator for up to three days.

VARIATION: Instead of the fresh Basil and roasted Garlic, just use 1/4–1/3 cup Garlic Galore Pesto (Rising Sun Farms Brand 800-888-0795). This is a lovely dairyless pesto that is also great on wraps. It is found in most large health-food stores.

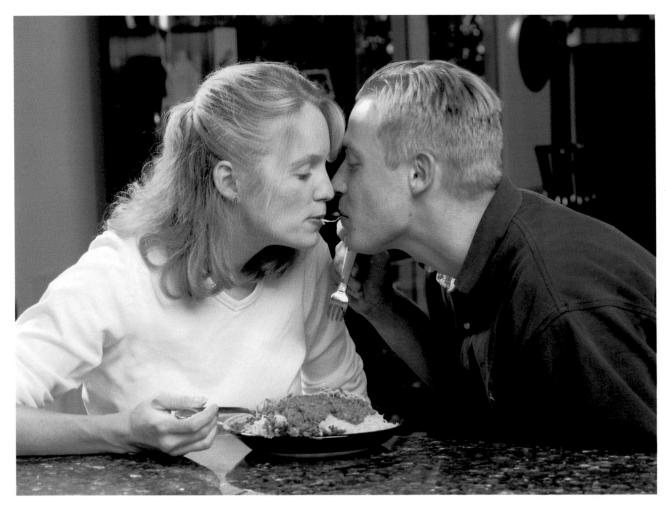

*See what fun you can have with Rich Raw Tomato Sauce!*

## Cauliflower Toss

*Serves 4.*

Layer half the lettuce and half the cauliflower in salad bowl. Top with radishes and remaining lettuce and cauliflower.

Mix dressing and pour over salad.

1/2 medium bunch Romaine Lettuce, torn
1/2 small head Cauliflower (broken into florets—2 cups)
1/4 cup Radishes, sliced

Dressing:
1/4 cup Flax Seed Oil
1 Green Onion, sliced
1/4 Tbs. dried Dill Weed
Vegetized Salt or Real Salt™
Freshly ground Pepper

## Rich Raw Tomato Sauce

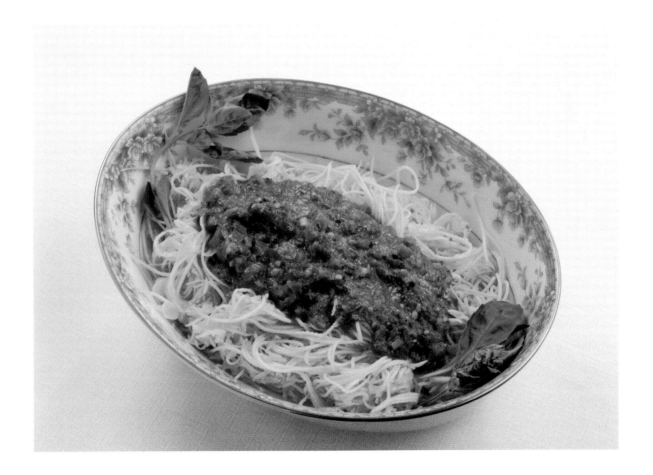

# Potassium Salad

1 part Cabbage
1 part Parsley
1 part Carrots

Dressing:
2/3 cup Flax Seed Oil
1/4 cup Bragg™ Liquid Aminos
Dulse, Garlic Powder, Onion Powder

Mix well.

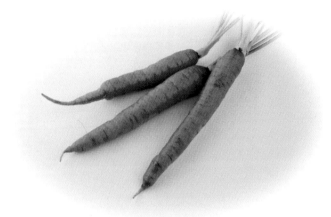

# Spiced Winter Squash

2 cups Butternut Squash, grated
2 Tbs. Olive Oil
1 cup grated Acorn or Banana Squash
2 tsp. Garam Masala or Curry (Spice Hunter)
Pinch of Cinnamon
1 Tbs. Lemon or Lime Juice or both
1 Tbs. Bragg™ Liquid Aminos
2 Tbs. minced Onion

Combine the squash, oil, spices, juice, Bragg™ Aminos, and onion. Mix well and toss. Then turn into an electric frypan and gently warm this dish right before serving.

# Three-Bean Salad

6 oz. steamed fresh Green Beans
6 oz. steamed fresh Wax Beans
6 oz. cooked Red Kidney Beans, drained
1/2 cup Green Onion, chopped
1/4 cup snipped fresh Parsley

Dressing:
1/4 cup Flax Seed Oil
1/8 cup Bragg™ Liquid Aminos
2 cloves Garlic, crushed
1/2 tsp. Italian Seasoning

Mix vegetables in large bowl.

Pour dressing over bean mixture, refrigerate 2 hours. Just before serving, remove bean mixture with slotted spoon onto lettuce bed.

# Bean Sprout Salad

*Serves 4.*

For dressing, combine oil, Liquid Aminos, pepper, garlic, and sesame seeds in blender, and purée. Rinse bean sprouts in cold water, and drain. In a bowl combine bean sprouts, pimento, and onion. Toss lightly in puréed dressing.

1/4 cup Flax Seed Oil
2 tsp. fresh Lemon Juice
2 Tbs. Bragg™ Liquid Aminos
1/2 tsp. freshly ground Pepper
2 Tbs. Sesame Seeds (soaked overnight)
1/4 cup Green Onion, finely chopped
1/4 cup Pimento, finely chopped
2 cups fresh Bean Sprouts
1 clove Garlic, crushed

# Alkalizing/Energizing Cucumber Salad

*Serves 3. Cucumber is one of the most alkalizing and energizing foods that you can eat. It is considered to have a purifying effect on the digestive system, and is very beneficial to the hair and skin. For a refreshing lift, lie down with a cucumber slice over each eye for a few minutes or rub a slice over your face after cleansing to tone and purify your skin.*

In a small serving bowl, combine the cucumbers, parsley, lemon juice, oil and mint. Toss together.

Chill for several hours or overnight. Toss again before serving.

2 cups Cucumbers, chopped
2 Tbs. Parsley, chopped
1 Tbs. Lemon Juice
1 Tbs. Flax Seed Oil or Olive Oil
1/3 cup finely chopped Peppermint

# Wheat Sprout Salad

*Serves 6.*

Mix all. Sprinkle with paprika. Serve on bed of lettuce.

3 cups fresh Wheat Sprouts (or any type of sprouts)
1 cup grated Carrots
3/4 cup minced Onion
3 Tbs. Flax Seed Oil
1 1/2 Tbs. fresh Lemon Juice

# Sprouted Lentil Salad

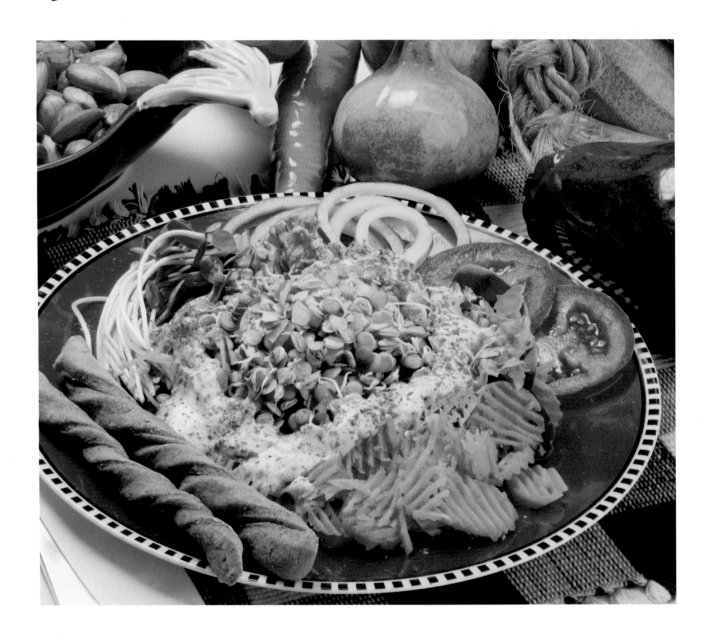

# Chilled Cucumber Refresher

*Serves 6.*

Combine broth and cucumber, chill, sprinkle each serving with dill weed.

4 cups yeast-free Vegetable Broth
1 cup Cucumber, shredded
Dill Weed

# Rainbow Salad

*I love the colors of vegetables! Presentation of a beautifully arranged alkalizing meal can be an art. This salad is my basic salad recipe that I make every week. The grating of the vegetables exposes so much of their natural sweetness. Serving the salad like this in a rainbow of colors is always pleasing to the eye. Enjoy with one of the many dressings in this Foundational Recipes section.*

*Eating a rainbow of colored foods is felt by some to support the balance of the energy of the body. By choosing foods of many colors, you are ensuring a wide variety of electrical/magnetic frequencies that will increase the level of energy in the body.*

Start with:
One big salad bowl with fresh, clean, dry greens (baby greens, spinach, lettuce, etc.).

Arrange the ingredients from the list on the top, going from the deepest dark colors to the lightest.

Top with a dressing of lemon juice and desired oil, with a sprinkle of sesame seeds.

Grated Red Cabbage
Grated Beets
Grated Carrots
Grated Squash (e.g., Butternut, Yellow Zucchini)
Grated Jicama
Red, Yellow, and Orange Bell Peppers
Sprouts
Cucumbers
Fresh Green Peas from the pod
Any thing else you want!

# Sprouted Lentil Salad

*Serves 4. This salad is hearty and also works well as a filling for halved bell peppers.*

In a small bowl, mix the oil, lemon juice, Liquid Aminos, garlic, "Zip," and curry powder. In a separate mixing bowl, combine the lentils and onions and toss.

Optional: Add some sprouted garbanzo beans, too!

2 cups sprouted Lentils
1/2 cup chopped Onions
1 Tbs. Lemon Juice
1 tsp. Bragg™ Liquid Aminos
1 tsp. Flax Seed Oil or Udo's Choice® Oil
1 clove Garlic, minced
1/2 chopped Onion
1 tsp. Curry Seasoning (Spice Hunter)
Pinch of "Zip" (Spice Hunter)

# Rainbow Salad

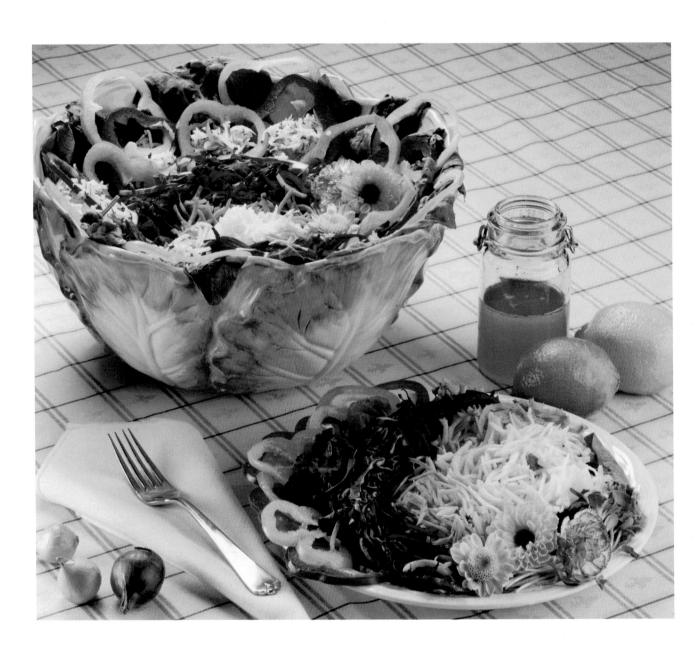

## Avocado/Tomato Snack

Blend all except tomatoes in blender until smooth. Spoon onto warmed tomato slices.

**2 Avocados**
**1 small Eggplant, diced**
**3/4 Tbs. Curry Powder**
**2 Tbs. Lemon Juice**
**2 Green Chili Peppers, seeded**
**Real Salt™ and seasoning to taste**
**2 or 3 Tomatoes, thickly sliced**

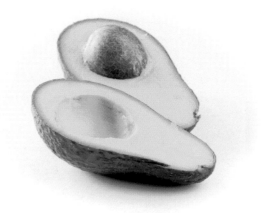

## Steam-Fried Sprouts

Steam-fry the onion and pepper in skillet, with Liquid Aminos. Add sprouts and steam gently for 30 seconds.

Serve immediately.

**2 Tbs. Bragg™ Liquid Aminos**
**2 cups fresh Bean Sprouts, any kind**
**1/2 cup Onion, finely chopped**
**1/2 cup Green or Red Pepper, finely chopped**

## Leprechaun Surprise Dip

Mix well. Serve with fresh vegetables.

**2 cups Spinach, very finely chopped**
**2 cups Parsley, very finely chopped**
**1 cup Green Onions, very finely chopped**
**1/2 cup Mock Mayo (see page 72)**

# Cinnamint Dressing

*This is a fresh tasting dressing that is not salty.*

**5 Tbs. Carrot Juice**
**1/2 cup Olive Oil**
**1/3 cup Lemon Juice**
**1 tsp. Orange Ginger Pepper blend (Spice Hunter)**
**1/2 tsp. Lemon Pepper**
**1/2 tsp. Cinnamon**
**1/8 tsp. Paprika**
**1 Tbs. fresh Mint, finely chopped**

Put all ingredients except mint in a food processor or blender. Blend until smooth. Stir in Mint.

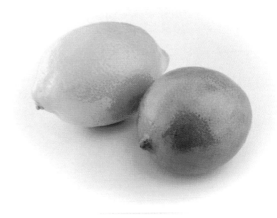

# Soy Cucumber Dressing

*A subtle refreshing dressing*

**2-3 tsp. Carrot Juice**
**1 lg. Cucumber (I prefer peeled and seeded)**
**1/2 Red Bell Pepper**
**1/2 small Onion**
**1 cup Soy Milk**
**1 tsp. dried Basil (or 2 tsp. fresh)**
**1 Tbs. Bragg™ Liquid Aminos or Real Salt™ to taste**

Blend all ingredients in food processor or blender until smooth.

# Flax Oil Dressing

**30% Flax Seed Oil**
**30% Bragg™ Liquid Aminos**
**40% Water**
**Liquid Lecithin to thicken and emulsify**
**Desired seasonings**

Blend briefly in blender, or shake and pour. Use as a dressing over salad or steamed veggies.

# Broccoli/Cauliflower Soup

In a food processor or blender, combine the almonds with the cucumber juice or broth, and garlic. Blend well. With machine still running, add the broccoli and cauliflower and blend until smooth. Lastly blend in seasonings and lemon/lime juice, Bragg™ Aminos, and salt. Add more broth or water to desired consistency.

Variation: Use an avocado instead of the almonds and use this recipe for a salad dressing.

1–2 cups Broccoli, chopped
1–2 cups Cauliflower, chopped
1 cup Cucumber Juice or Veggie Broth (Pacific brand)
1/2 cup soaked Almonds
1 clove Garlic, minced
1/4 tsp. Cumin
1/4 tsp. Curry Powder
1 Tbs. Lemon or Lime Juice
1 Tbs. Bragg™ Liquid Aminos
1/2 tsp. Real Salt™

# Creamy Vegetable Soup

*This rich soup gets its creaminess from tofu. Be sure to blend it thoroughly (I think the blender is best) so you get a rich, even, smooth, creamy texture. Serves 10.*

In a skillet, steam-fry the onions and garlic for a few minutes. Add cabbage, celery, and asparagus. Transfer to a large pot, add the leeks and vegetable broth. Stir in the parsley, dill, basil, oregano, salt, and pepper. Simmer just to brighten veggies. Let cool a bit, then purée in a blender or food processor two cups at a time with some of the tofu, and return to another pot. Heat soup, not to exceed 118°, and serve.

1 cup Onion, chopped
2 cloves Garlic, minced
2 large Leeks, chopped
3 Celery Stalks, chopped
2 cups shredded Green Cabbage
1/2 lb. Asparagus, cut small
1 pkg. soft FRESH Tofu
4 cups Vegetable Broth
2 Tbs. chopped fresh Parsley
2 tsp. dried Dill, 2 tsp. dried Basil, 1 tsp. dried Oregano
Real Salt™ and Pepper to taste

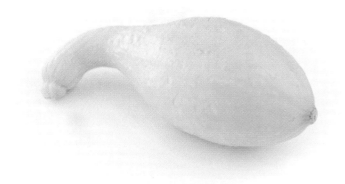

# Alfalfa Sprout Salad

*Serves 6.*

3 cups Alfalfa Sprouts
3 cups Summer Squash, chopped
2 Red Peppers, diced
2 Green Onions, chopped
1/4 cup Seed Onion, chopped

Dressing:
Flax Seed Oil, fresh Lemon Juice, Real Salt™

# Popeye Mousse Pie

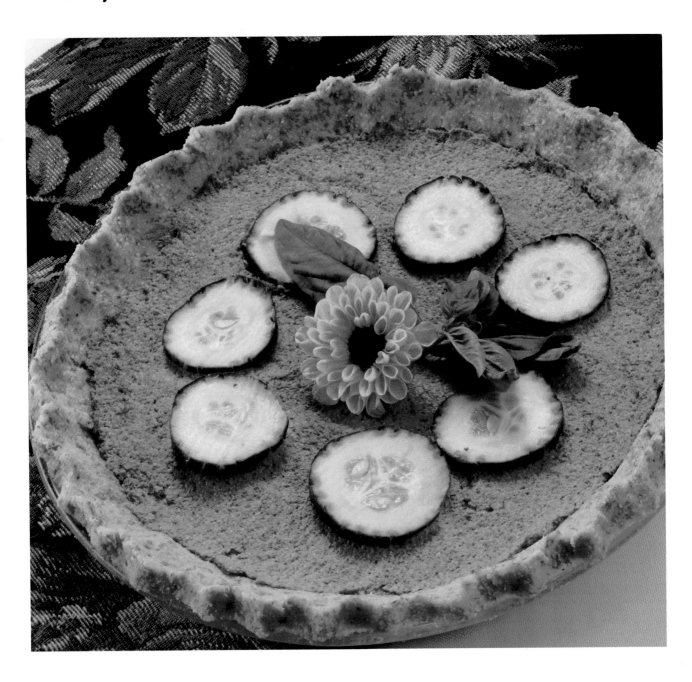

# Popeye Mousse Pie

*This recipe uses psyllium seed powder to act as the binding agent that helps it set up. Ask your health food store for this item or you can buy psyllium seed and grind it into a powder in a small coffee grinder. Makes one 9-inch pie.*

For the crust, process the nuts in your food processor until they are uniformly fine. Add the Liquid Aminos and pulse-chop. Gradually add the water until mixture holds together. Finally sprinkle the psyllium and seasoning while the processor is running. Press into a 9-inch pan and set aside.

For the mousse, put in the food processor the spinach, lemon juice, Liquid Aminos, and water, and process until smooth. Add the tahini, onion, and dill. Process until the mixture is a thick purée. Gradually sprinkle in the psyllium while the machine is running. Press the paté into the pie crust immediately. Refrigerate for at least 30 minutes or up to 24 hours before eating.

**Almond Crust:**
2–3 cups Almonds, soaked 8–12 hours
1 Tbs. Bragg™ Liquid Aminos
2–4 Tbs. Water or Lemon Juice
1 Tbs. Psyllium Powder
1 tsp. Garlic Herb Bread Seasoning (Spice Hunter)

**Popeye Mousse:**
5 cups coarsely chopped Spinach
1/2 cups raw Pine Nuts
1/3–1/2 cup Lemon Juice
1 Tbs. Bragg™ Liquid Aminos
1 Tbs. Water
1/2 cup firm Tofu
1 Tbs. Red Onion, chopped
1 Tbs. freshly chopped Dill, or 1 1/2 tsp. Deliciously Dill spice (Spice Hunter)
1 stalk Celery, coarsely chopped
2 tsp. Psyllium Powder

# Celery/Cauliflower Soup

1. Steam-fry the onion in a little water in a large soup pan for about 5 minutes without browning. Pulse-chop the celery and cauliflower in the food processor until finely chopped.

2. Add the celery and cauliflower mix to the pan and warm until tender. Add the vegetable stock, almond milk, and simmer for about 15–30 minutes, or you can leave this raw and not cook at all.

3. Purée the soup mixture in a blender or food processor until smooth texture is achieved. Season with salt and other seasonings of choice. Serve warm or cold.

1 Onion peeled and chopped
1 whole head Celery, trimmed and chopped (save some celery leaves for garnish)
1 head Cauliflower, trimmed and chopped
1 Tbs. Oil (Olive or Udo's)
1–2 quarts Vegetable Stock
1/2–1 quarts Almond Milk
Salt, Pepper, and Seasonings of choice to taste.

61

# Casserole de Cauliflower

*Serves 4-6. 20 minutes to prepare. This dish is a lot like couscous in texture and makes a great breakfast, lunch, or dinner side dish.*

2 tsp. Oil (Olive, Flax, or Udo's Choice®)
2–4 tsp. Cumin
1–2 tsp. Turmeric
1/2 Yellow or Red Onion, finely minced
1 cup Water
Flowerets from 1 very large or 2 small Cauliflowers
4 Tbs. fresh Parsley, minced
1/2 cup raw Pine Nuts
7–8 Sun-dried Tomatoes (Melissa's brand are packed in olive oil)
Bragg™ Liquid Aminos to taste
Lemon or Lime Juice to taste
2 cloves Garlic, minced

1. In an electric skillet, warm the oil, cumin, and turmeric.

2. Keeping the temperature on warm or low, add the onion and allow the flavors to blend for 2–4 minutes, then add the water and warm.

3. In a food processor fitted with an S-blade, process the cauliflower into very small pieces (like couscous). Also process the sun-dried tomatoes into fine small pieces.

4. Add the cauliflower to the skillet and gradually warm, adding the parsley, bell pepper, garlic, sun-dried tomatoes and pine nuts. Season with Bragg™ Aminos to taste. Enjoy!

# Fresh Cucumber Dills

*Serves 6.*

2 large Cucumbers, peeled and thinly sliced
Stir Together:
2 Tbs. fresh Dill Weed
1 Tbs. fresh Lemon Juice
3 Tbs. distilled Water
1/2 tsp. Real Salt™
Dash of Cayenne Pepper

Drain cucumbers well, add dressing. Stir in well.

Cover and chill overnight.

# Fresh Spinach Filling

1 1/2 cups finely chopped fresh Spinach
3 Tbs. Mock Mayo (see p. 62)
1 Tbs. chopped Pimento
1/4 tsp. Onion Powder
1 tsp. fresh Lemon Juice

Otherwise season to taste. Delicious in sprouted wheat tortillas.

# Casserole de Cauliflower

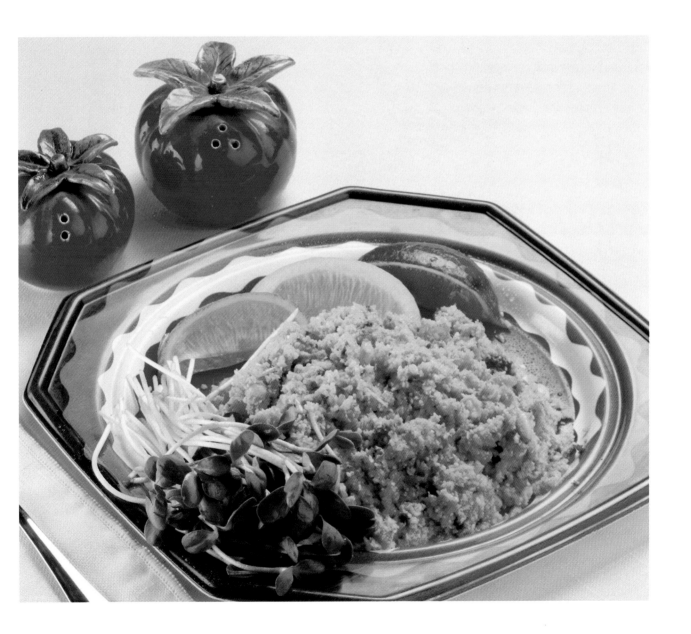

## Maren's Salsa

6 cloves minced Garlic
Finely chop:
1 yellow Onion
1/2  cup fresh Cilantro
1/2  cup fresh Parsley
7 ripe Tomatoes
1 Green Pepper
1 Red Pepper
Juice of 1 Lemon and 1 Lime (about 10 Tbs.)
Real Salt™ to taste
Mexican Seasoning (Spice Hunter) to taste
Cajun Seasoning by Tones to taste
Cayenne Pepper and Cumin to taste

Blend together and refrigerate.

# *Mock Mayo*

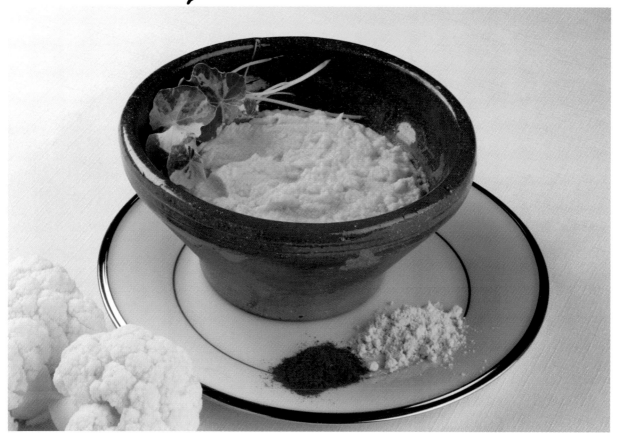

# Tofu Salad Spread

*Yield: 3 1/2 cups.*

Mix all ingredients. Serve on a bed of greens.

8 oz. FRESH Tofu, well drained (I use Nigari)
3/4 cup chopped Green Onion
1 cup Celery, finely chopped
3/4 cup Carrot, finely chopped
6 Tbs. Mock Mayo (see below)
1 Tbs. dried Parsley
1/4 tsp. each of Basil, Sage, Thyme
1 1/2 tsp. Vegetized Salt or Real Salt™
1/2 tsp. Garlic Powder
1/8 tsp. Cayenne Pepper

# Mock Mayo

Whip the cauliflower with a little water and flax seed oil, and add the remaining ingredients.

1 cup steamed Cauliflower
1/4 tsp. Real Salt™
1/4 tsp. dry Mustard
1/4 tsp. Paprika
Cayenne Pepper to taste
1/2–1 tsp. oil (Udo's) to emulsify

# Mock Almond Mayonnaise

In a food processor or blender combine the almonds with water or broth and process until smooth. Add lemon, onion, red pepper, garlic, oil, oregano, Liquid Aminos, and spices. Blend until smooth, using additional water if necessary to achieve the desired consistency. This can be a great dressing for salad or a dip with dehydrated veggies added. Enjoy!

1 cup soaked Almonds
1/2 cup Water or Veggie Broth
1 Tbs. dried Onion or 3 Tbs. chopped Onion
3 Tbs. chopped Red Pepper
1 clove Garlic
1 Lemon, peeled and chopped
1 Tbs. Oil (Udo's Choice® or Flax Seed Oil)
1 tsp. dried Oregano, or 1 Tbs. fresh
2 tsp. Dulse flakes
2 tsp. Bragg™ Liquid Aminos
Pinch each of Cumin, Curry Seasoning, and "Zip"

# Crispy Radish Filling

3/4 cup finely chopped Celery
1/2 cup finely chopped Radishes
4 Tbs. Mock Mayo (see p.62)
1 Tbs. chopped Chives
1/4 tsp. Real Salt™
Few grains of Pepper

Great for stuffing celery, on sprouted wheat bread or sprouted wheat tortilla roll-ups.

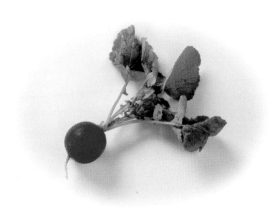

# Garden Variety Filling

3/4 cup grated Carrot
1/2 cup finely chopped Celery
2 Tbs. grated Jalapeño Soy Cheese
3 Tbs. Mock Mayo (see p. 62)
1 Tbs. finely chopped Green Pepper
1 Tbs. Bragg™ Liquid Aminos
1/4 tsp. Real Salt™
1/4 tsp. Cayenne Pepper
Few grains of Black Pepper

Excellent to stuff celery sticks or with vegetables.

# Garbanzo Spread

*Yield: 3 cups.*

2 cups sprouted, cooked or raw Garbanzo
 Beans (Chickpeas)
1 med. Onion, chopped
2 Tbs. dried Parsley
1 tsp. Real Salt™
1 tsp. Coriander
Dash Cayenne or Chili Powder
1/4 cup Water

Blend all in blender until smooth. Spread on sprouted whole wheat tortillas, topped with alfalfa sprouts, or eat with veggies.

# Garden Variety Filling

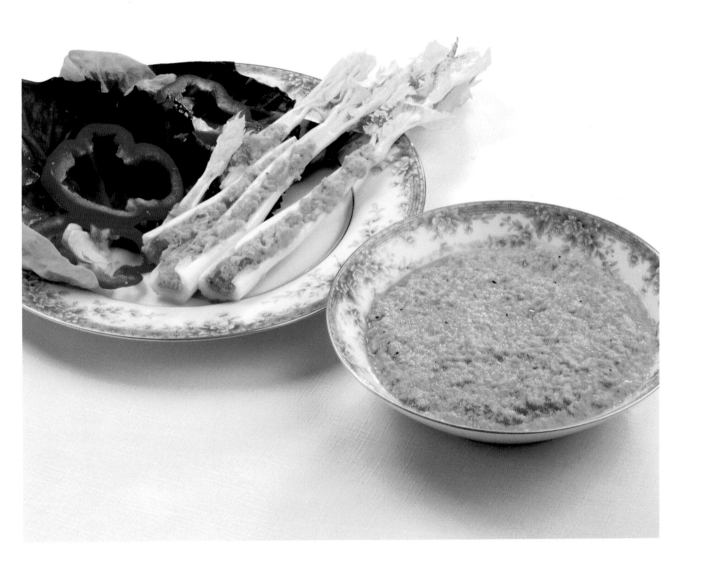

# Herbed Salad Dressing

1 tsp. dry Mustard
1 tsp. fresh Parsley
1 tsp. Dill Weed
1/2 tsp. Real Salt™
1/4 tsp. Tarragon
1/4 tsp. ground Black Pepper
1/8 tsp. Thyme
1/3 cup preferred oil (Virgin Olive, Grape Seed, Udo's, or Flax Seed)
Pinch of Oregano

# Spicy Asian Dressing

*This dressing is easily whipped up in the food processor and gives your salads a wonderful Asian Zing. If you tend not to like too much spice, then half the amounts of spices listed..*

1/3 cup + 1 Tbs. Sesame Tahini
1/2 cup Water
1/2 cup Braggs
2 tsp. dried Onions
6 Tbs. Flaxseed Oil
1/2–1 tsp. Chicory Root Powder (sweetener)
3 Tbs. Grated Ginger Root
1/2 tsp. Chinese 5 Spice Seasoning
1/8–1/4 tsp. Cayenne Pepper or Hot Zip (Spice Hunter)
1/2 tsp. Cumin
Optional: Add water to thin if needed

Place all ingredients in food processor and process until smooth and well mixed. This dressing will last several days in the refrigerator.

# Herb Oil

*Yield: 3/4 cup.*

1/2 cup Flax Seed Oil, Olive Oil, or Udo's
2 Tbs. Lemon Juice
1/2 tsp. Real Salt™
1/8 tsp. freshly ground Black Pepper
1/4 cup finely chopped fresh Parsley
1/2 tsp. dried Tarragon Leaves
Dash of Cayenne Pepper

Mix all ingredients well. Store in jar, refrigerate. Great on salads, steamed veggies.

# Herbed Salad Dressing

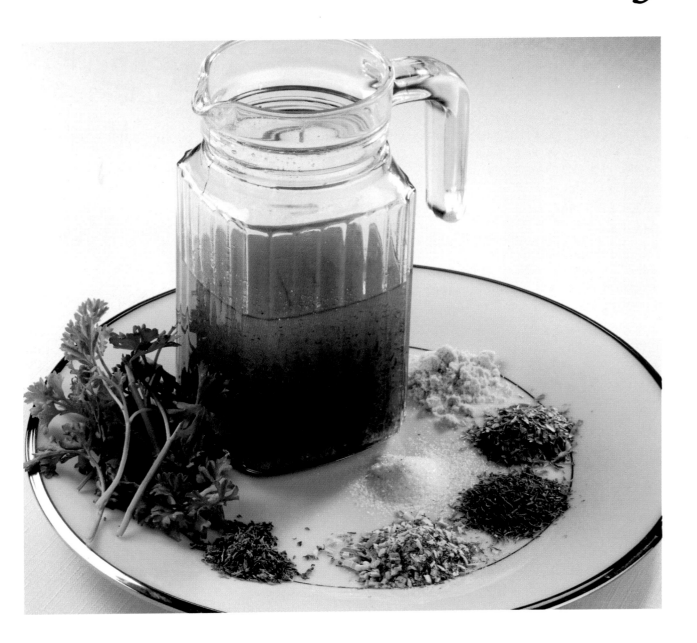

# Essential Dressing

50% Flax Seed Oil or Hemp Oil

50% Bragg™ Liquid Aminos (you may want to dilute)

Liquid Lecithin to emulsify

Parsley flakes and/or other seasoning, such as kelp

# Curried Carrot Almond Dressing

*This dressing is simple, fast and full of great flavor. I have found that it is best if you first blanch the soaked almonds to remove their skins. Since this dressing has fresh carrot juice in it, it is highly perishable, so make only enough to use up in one or two days.*

1/2 cup Almonds, soaked and blanched with skins removed (a rubber garlic cylinder roller takes the skins off fast).

1 cup fresh Carrot Juice

1/3 to 1/2 tsp. Curry Powder

1/2 tsp. dried Onion

Squirt of Bragg™ to taste

Dash of Lemon or Lime Juice to taste

Optional: 1 clove fresh or 2 cloves roasted garlic

Put all ingredients in a blender and blend at high speed until smooth. If you want this for more of a dip, then use more almonds and less carrot juice, and process to desired thickness.

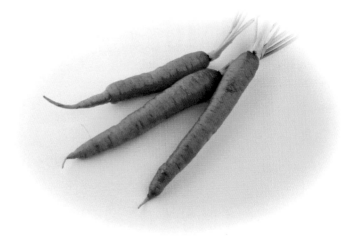

# Parsley Dressing

1 3/4 cups Water

2 Celery Stalks

1/3 cup preferred oil (Virgin Olive, Grape Seed, Udo's, or Flax Seed Oil)

1–3 cloves Garlic

1/4 cup Parsley

Optional: Salt or other Seasonings of choice

Blend together all ingredients. Use on salad, veggies.

# Tahini Dressing/Dip

Put all ingredients in food processor and blend until smooth. Thin with water/oil for dressing, or let set up in the fridge for a dip.

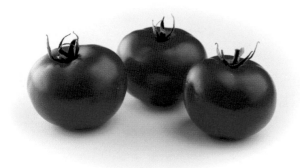

1 cup Raw Tahini
1 tsp. dried Parsley or 1/2 cup fresh Parsley
1 Tbs. dried Onion or 1 small Onion, chopped
2 tsp. Tomato Powder (order thru Robert O. Young Research Center 801-756-7850)
2 tsp. Cucumber powder
1 fresh Tomato, chopped
2 Tbs. Lemon/Lime juice (I use more)
1 tsp. fresh Cilantro, finely chopped
1/2 tsp. Cumin
1–3 cloves Garlic or 4–6 cloves roasted Garlic
Shot of Bragg™ to taste
1 tsp. Real Salt™
Pinch of Cayenne or "Zip"

# Ginger/Almond Dressing

In a food processor, process the scallions, ginger, and garlic until smooth. Add almond butter, oil, Liquid Aminos, and process until the mixture is blended. Slowly add the water to desired consistency, and continue processing until well blended. Serve on non-starchy veggies, salads, etc.

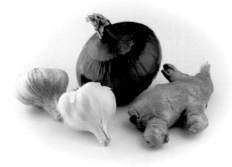

3 Scallions (white part only)
Peeled fresh Ginger (thin, 2-inch slice)
2 Garlic cloves
4 Tbs. Almond Butter
1 tsp. Flax Seed Oil
Bragg™ Liquid Aminos to taste
1–2 cups Water
Optional: 1 tsp. dehydrated vegetable powder (I use tomato) or 1–2 sundried tomatoes packed in olive oil.

# Basic Seasoning Recipe

Mix all ingredients together. Store in a tightly capped jar and use as a vegetable seasoning.

1 1/2 oz. Onion Powder
1/2 oz. Garlic Powder
2 oz. Comfrey Leaf or Celery Leaf Powder, or mixture
1/2 tsp. Red Cayenne Pepper
1 tsp. powdered Kelp
1/2 oz. Ginger Root Powder

# Lime Ginger Sauce

*This makes a wonderful sauce, dressing, or marinade.*

1/4 cup Lime Juice

1/4 cup Oil (Flax Seed Oil, Olive Oil, or Udo's Choice®)

1 Tbs. Bragg™ Liquid Aminos

1/4 cup Water

1 Tbs. fresh Mint

1 Tbs. fresh Cilantro

1 tsp. minced Ginger Root

1/4 tsp. dried Red Chili Pepper

2–3 tsp. fresh Jicama or Carrot Juice

1 tsp. Real Salt™ to taste

Dash of "Zip"

In a processor or blender combine all ingredients and blend well.

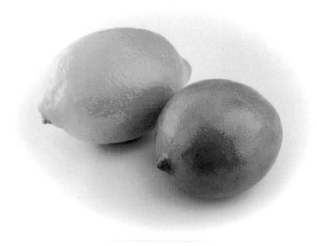

# Wowie Zowie Almond Butter Dressing

*This is a rich sweet dressing that tastes great on salads, over rice, or on top of any steamed veggies. Children will especially like this dressing because of it's creamy nut butter taste.  Add additional water to thin if desired.*

1 cup Raw Almond Butter (I use Marantha Brand)

1/2–1 cup Water

Juice of 1 Lemon

1 Tbs. Bragg™ or 1 tsp. Real Salt™

2 tsp. Chicory Root powder (sweetener)

1 heaping Tbs. Dried Onion

2 cloves Garlic

1 Tbs. grated Fresh Ginger Root

1 Tbs. Sesame Oil

1/2 tsp. Zip (Spice Hunter)

In a blender or food processor, combine almond butter, water, lemon juice, Braggs,  and Chicory Root. After this is well blended leave blender on and add the onion, garlic, ginger, oil, and zip. Blend well and add additional water if required for thinner consistency. Can be served warmed or cool. Enjoy!

# CHAPTER 5

# Framework

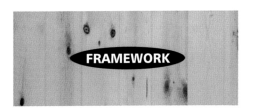

FRAMEWORK

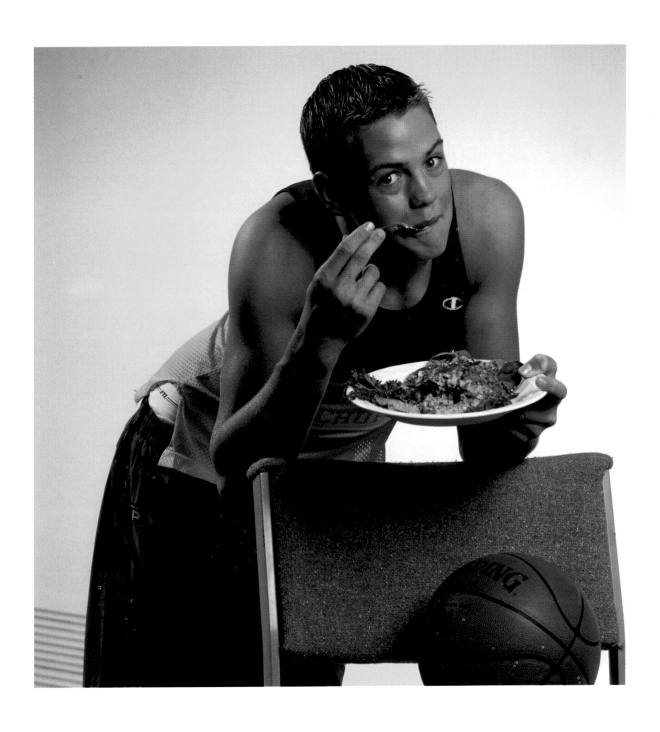

*Nothing will benefit human health and increase the chances for survival of life on earth as much as the evolution to a vegetarian diet.*

**—Albert Einstein**

## Entrées and Side Dishes

These are recipes to use as your health becomes more balanced. After you have decided on the 70–80 percent alkalizing part of your meal, these framework recipes can be added to make up the other 20–30 percent of your meal. Some of these recipes are warmed, processed, or cooked, therefore they will require more time to digest and may offer some grounding effects to a meal. The framework recipes would not normally be eaten while on a cleanse or when experiencing an acute illness or imbalance in the body. After the cleanse and the first 8 to 12 weeks of eating very alkaline, when a balance in the internal terrain has been established, then the framework recipes can be added. (For information on cleansing and rebalancing, refer to Dr. Young's Complete Program and Diet™, through the Robert O. Young Research Center, 801-756-7850.) Special care and observation of symptoms should be noted as the framework foods are added back into the diet. If symptoms return, then perhaps a longer period of totally alkalizing meals would be in order until more healing takes place.

Framework recipes add more texture and important variety to a meal and also help tremendously when someone is transitioning from high-acid foods. They are great recipes to use when helping children to phase off from meat, dairy, and sugars. Again, enjoy this journey of new substitutes in your nutritional choices. After a while, these framework recipes will become like second nature, and you will look forward to serving them to your family and everyone you entertain. Bon Appetit!

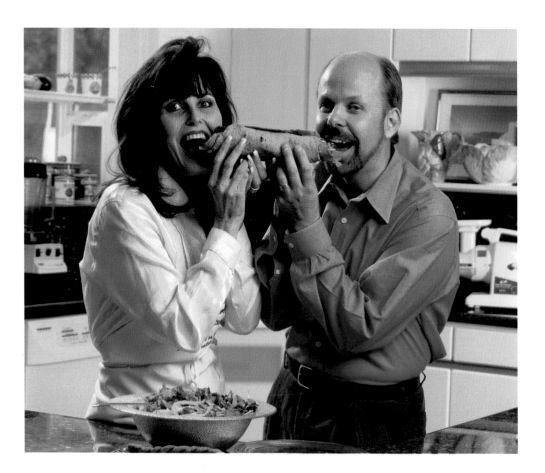

# Mexicali Rice

*This is a salsa rice that is a great complement to a Mexican dinner. Serve with Great Olé Guacamole and Green Chili Tofu Pita Hors D'oeuvres.*

Put half the olive oil in a skillet or electric frypan, and sauté the onion and garlic until onion softens. Then add the rest of the ingredients (I chop them all up in a food processor) and steam-fry until veggies are bright and still somewhat crisp. Add 3–4 cups cooked rice and the rest of the olive oil. Mix well and serve warm.

3 Tbs. Olive Oil
1 Onion, chopped
1/2 cup Celery, diced
1/4 cup Bell Pepper, diced
1 clove Garlic, minced
2 large Tomatoes, coarsely chopped
2 Serrano Chilies, seeds and stems removed, chopped
2 Tbs. fresh Cilantro, chopped
1 tsp. fresh Lime Juice
1/2 tsp. Oregano
1 tsp. Real Salt™

# Shelley's Super Tortillas

Mix all ingredients in a food processor with a dough S-blade. Use the pulse-chop action to prevent overheating the motor. When the dough forms into one big ball, turn out onto a floured flat surface and break off balls and roll them out to about 1/8–1/4-inch thickness. Transfer to an electric pan that has been lightly oiled, and heat on both sides until you see a few air pockets rise. Take off the burner and let cool, then wrap in an air-tight bag and keep in the fridge or freezer. Do not overcook, unless you want a crisped tortilla to use with dips or soups.

If you can find dehydrated vegetable powders, you can add them for color and flavor. (Dr. Young has created a whole line of vegetable powders, a concentrate of 20–1, e.g., spinach, parsley, broccoli, cabbage, tomato, celery, carrot, beet, etc.) For information on the vegetable powders, contact the Robert O. Young Research Center to order (801) 756-7850. Or you can decrease the milk or water and add fresh vegetable juices instead, like spinach, parsley or carrot.

4 cups Flour (use any mix of flours you like, such as whole wheat, unbleached white, spelt, etc.)
2 tsp. Real Salt™
2–4 tsp. of concentrated Vegetable Powders (I use tomato and celery a lot)
4 tsp. Seasonings of your choice (I use Spice Hunter's Mexican and California Pizza)
2 Tbs. dried Onions
12 Sun-dried Tomatoes (packed in olive oil)
2 tsp. Garlic powder
2–4 leaves fresh Basil
1 1/2 cups Coconut Milk or Water
2 Tbs. Olive Oil

# Shelley's Super Wraps

*Wraps are today's answer to healthy fast food. If you stock your refrigerator with some "basics," you can make a wrap in just a few minutes. They travel well, and if you include your favorite spices, they can be "to-die-for" delicious!*

**Soaked Almonds**

**Sun-dried Tomatoes (bottled in olive oil)**

**Red, Yellow, Orange or Green Peppers**

**Raw Veggies: Carrots, Broccoli, Cauliflower, etc.**

**Red Onions**

**Roasted Garlic**

**Sprouts**

**Pine Nuts**

**Top with Lemon or Lime Juice**

**Add your favorite spices**

I start with a tortilla, either one made from the Super Tortillas recipe, or you can use a sprouted wheat tortilla from the health food store. Sometimes you can get a "wrap" café or restaurant to sell you their tortillas and can keep them in the freezer or fridge. You can also find great hummus and non-dairy pesto at your local health food store.

Lay out your tortilla flat and spread with non-dairy pesto or hummus, or any spread you like. The Roasted Pepper Macadamia Sauce (see page 79) or even the Raw Pecan Paté (see page 113) also work well.

Then lay several leaves of romaine lettuce down the center. You could also use any other lettuce or even mixed green salad. On top of the green lettuce place any of the ingredient items.:

Then roll up the wrap and secure tightly in saran wrap (a couple of layers). Eat immediately, or at least within the same day, as the tortilla can become soggy. Enjoy!

# Nepal Vegetable Curry

*Serves 4–6.*

**1 Onion, chopped**

**1 Bay Leaf, broken**

**1 Green Chili, chopped**

**1 clove Garlic, minced**

**1 inch Ginger, grated**

**1/4 tsp. Turmeric**

**Real Salt™ or Vegetized Salt to taste**

**1 lb. Carrots, cubed**

**1/2 Cauliflower, broken into florets**

**1 cup Green Peas**

**1 tsp. each, Coriander and Cumin**

**1 cup hot Water**

Lightly steam-fry onion. Add bay leaf, chili, garlic, ginger, turmeric, salt. Stir in carrots and sauté lightly. Add remaining ingredients and hot water. Cook gently on medium heat until vegetables are tender.

# Shelley's Super Wraps

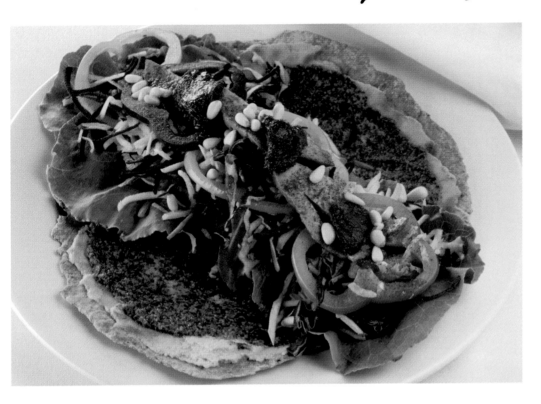

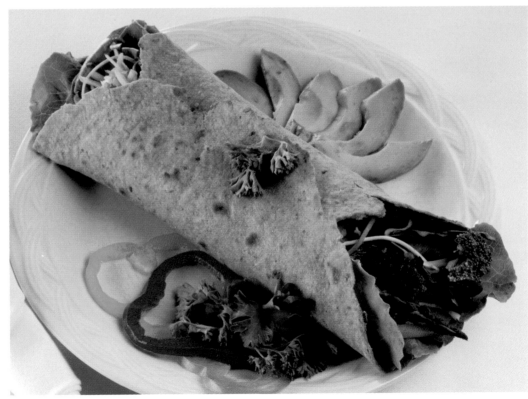

# Tofu Italian Mock Meatballs

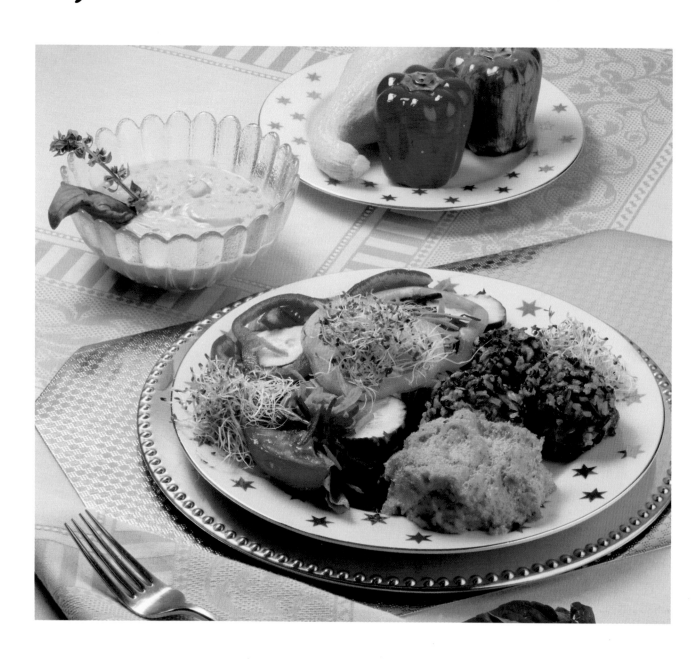

# Tofu Italian Mock Meatballs

*Makes 10 two-inch or 40 one-inch balls. This is a great transitional food when phasing off from meat. If wild rice is used, a sweet nutty flavor will result. They can be served warm for a main course, and also make a great cool snack right out of the fridge. (We always double this recipe because everyone loves them!)*

1. Take 8–10 sprouted wheat tortillas and leave them out to dry on a counter or quick-dry them in a low-heat oven. Break them into small pieces and blend in a Vita-Mix® or food processor until they are finely ground into crumbs. Set aside in a bowl.

2. In an electric skillet, steam-fry the celery, onion, garlic, and cook until softened, about 6 minutes. Transfer to a large bowl. Put the tofu, vegetable stock, oats, and Liquid Aminos in a blender and blend until smooth. Add the parsley, basil, black pepper, and "Zip," and pulse until well blended. Add to the onion mixture.

3. Add the cooked wild rice to the onion mixture, along with the tortilla crumbs, and mix well. Mixture should be slightly sticky but form into balls easily. You may need to add more tortilla crumbs if mixture is too wet.

4. Preheat oven to 400°. Lightly oil a baking dish or cookie sheet. Shape mixture into balls, and roll each ball into the remaining tortilla crumbs to coat. Bake until lightly browned, 20–30 minutes. Serve with Roasted Pepper Macadamia Sauce sauce to dip the balls in. Enjoy!

1 cup cooked Brown and Wild Rice, 50/50
2 stalks Celery with leaves, finely chopped
1 med. Red Onion, finely chopped
2 cloves Garlic, minced
2 lbs. FIRM Tofu (Nigari), crumbled
1 cup Vegetable Stock (Pacific Foods of Oregon brand)
1/4 cup whole Rolled Oats
3 Tbs. Bragg™ Liquid Aminos
2 cups fresh Basil, finely chopped
2 cups Parsley
1/4 tsp. Black Pepper, freshly ground
2 tsp. "Zip" or pinch of Cayenne Pepper
1–2 cups Sprouted Wheat Tortilla crumbs
1 Tbs. Olive Oil
Spice Hunter's Herbes de Provence to taste (about 1 tsp.)

# Roasted Pepper Macadamia Sauce

*This is a rich beautifully colored sauce that can be made thick for dipping with grilled Tofu slices or the Tofu Mock Meatballs, or it can be thinned and used as a WOW salad dressing.*

Put all ingredients except oil in a food processor and process until creamy, then slowly add olive oil until well emulsified.

4–5 big pieces of roasted Red Peppers (you can roast them or buy bottled)
6 cloves roasted Garlic
1 lb. Macadamia Nuts (raw is best, roasted will give a different flavor)
1/2 to 1 cup Olive Oil
3 large fresh Basil Leaves
Real Salt™ and Pepper to taste

# Cabbage Stuffed Vegetables

8 Cabbage Leaves

1 cup French-Style Green Beans

3 tsp. dehydrated Onion Flakes moistened
    with Tomato Juice or Veggie Broth

2 stalks Celery

1/2 cup Bean Sprouts

1/2 Green Bell Pepper

1 tsp. Parsley (chopped)

2 cups Vegetable Broth

Scald cabbage leaves with boiling water and leave covered in pot for one-half hour. Chop all vegetables fine, add parsley and mix. Spoon vegetable mixture onto each cabbage leaf. Roll tight and tuck in ends. Fasten with toothpicks, simmer in vegetable broth for 1 hour. Serve, season with Braggs™ Liquid Aminos, flax seed oil, and cayenne pepper.

# Cajun-Style Red Beans and Brown Rice

*Yield: 9 servings.   Per serving; 1 cup beans, 2/3 cup rice.*

1 lb. dried Pinto Beans

2 cups Yellow Onion (chopped)

1 cup Green Onions (chopped)

1 cup Green Bell Pepper (chopped)

1/2 tsp. Garlic (minced)

1/4 tsp. Red Cayenne Pepper

3/4 tsp. Black Pepper

1/2 tsp Celtic Sea Salt

1/4 tsp. Oregano

1/4 tsp. Garlic Powder

1 oz. Braggs™ Liquid Aminos

4 Tbs. Cayenne Pepper

6 oz. Tomato Paste

1/4 tsp. Thyme

1 tsp. Celery Flakes

6 cups cooked Brown Rice

1. Wash beans and then soak for 12 hours.

2. Drain water.

3. Fill a large pot with beans, add water to 1/2" above beans.

4. Add remaining ingredients, cook over low heat 2 to 2 1/2 hours, covered.

5. Serve over cooked brown rice.

# Stuffed Acorn Squash

2 small Acorn Squash, halved and seeded

1/2 cup Onion, diced

1/2 cup Carrot, diced

1/2 cup Red Bell Pepper, diced

1/2 cup Zucchini, thickly sliced

1/2 tsp. minced Garlic

Non-Stick Vegetable Spray

Preheat oven to 350°. Spray a large baking dish with cooking spray. Steam acorn squash halves by placing cut sides down in pan with 1/4 cup water for 10 to 15 minutes. Lightly steam-fry remaining ingredients, a few minutes only, stirring frequently. Spoon vegetables into squash halves. Bake 20–25 minutes or until squash is tender.

# Green Chili Tofu Pita Hors D'oeuvres

*These are great little Mexican Triangles stuffed with a fresh tofu/cilantro filling. Great for a snack or as a main course beside a big salad.*

1. Take the pita bread and cut it like a pie into eight triangular pieces and open each one up so you can put the filling in. In a food processor mince the garlic, then add all other ingredients except the tofu, and process until finely chopped. Then put the grater attachment on the processor and grate the tofu into the mix. Process for a few seconds more to mix.

2. Spoon the filling into the pita triangles and place into a pie pan. Spoon enchilada sauce over each pita and inside over the filling mixture. Bake at 350° for 10–15 minutes. Cut sun-dried tomatoes and avocado slices to put on top for a garnish just before serving warm.

1 pkg. Pita Bread or Tortillas

1 small can Green Chilies (chopped)

3 cloves Garlic, minced

1 pkg. extra firm Tofu (Nigari)

1 tsp. Mexican Seasoning (Spice Hunter)

2 tsp. dried Onion, OR 1/4 cup minced fresh Onion

1/4 cup Soy Parmesan Cheese substitute

1 Tbs. fresh Cilantro

1/2 tsp. Real Salt™

1 jar or can Enchilada Sauce

Avocado slices for garnish

3–4 Sun-dried Tomatoes for garnish

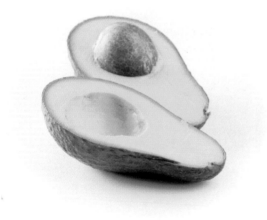

# Kale with Egyptian Garlic Sauce

*Makes 2 or 3 side-dish servings. Kale is a tasty green and deserves to be better known. Its ruffled leaves cook to a deep green and appealing accompaniment for rice or other whole grains. Kale is delicious with an Egyptian sauce of sautéed garlic and ground coriander. It's not exactly a sauce, but a seasoning mixture—a way to add a quick burst of flavor to a cooked vegetable; also good with okra or baked eggplant. It can also be mixed with brown rice and zucchini.*

Rinse kale and remove stems, including the tough part of stem in the leaf. Pile leaves and cut into manageable size. Steam kale until tender-crisp, and transfer to a bowl. Steam-fry garlic, about 1 minute. Add coriander, salt, and cayenne and stir over low heat for 15 seconds to blend. Immediately toss with kale, in pan or in a bowl. Taste and adjust seasoning. Serve hot.

1 lb. Kale

2 tsp. ground Coriander

4 med. Garlic cloves, minced

Real Salt™ and Cayenne Pepper

# Autumn Curry Crepes with Curried Veggie Filling

*This wonderfully colorful Thai-tasting dish can be served as an hors d'oeuvre snack, or as a side dish to your main course. Serve the crepes fresh from the grill, as you make them, or save them in the fridge and fill them the next morning for a really spicy warm breakfast!*

1 cup Almond Milk (I use Pacific brand)

3 Tbs. unsweetened Coconut Milk

1/2 tsp. Turmeric

1/4 tsp. Curry Powder

Dash of Cinnamon

1 1/2 tsp. Egg Replacer OR 1 1/2 Tbs. Agar Agar flakes (seaweed gel, found in your health food store)

1/3 cup Water

1 Tbs. Olive Oil

1 cup all-purpose Flour (or spelt, millet, or whole wheat flour)

1/2 tsp. Salt (optional)

1. In a bowl, whisk together the almond milk, coconut milk, egg replacer or agar agar flakes, water, oil, turmeric, cinnamon, and curry. Then whisk in the flour and salt until there are no lumps left in the batter. If you are using agar agar, then put the mixture in a food processor and process until smooth. Put saran wrap over the bowl and refrigerate for at least one-half hour or up to one day.

2. Heat a small nonstick crepe pan or skillet (I use my electric frypan) over medium-low heat. If batter has begun to separate, gently stir it to blend back in again. Once the pan is hot, drop 2 Tbs. of crepe batter into the skillet and swirl the pan to coat the bottom evenly with the batter. If the batter does not swirl easily, add a little water to thin it down a bit. Cook the crepe until the top appears dry, about a minute or two. Using a spatula, gently flip the crepe, and cook until the bottom appears lightly browned and the crepe slides easily in the pan, about a minute or two more. Transfer the crepe to a paper towel or plate. The crepes may be made in advance and refrigerated or frozen.

# Curried Veggie Filling

*This filling is spicy and colorful! You can substitute veggies of your choice and it always come out tasty! This dish is especially good in the autumn or winter because of its warming spices and grounding effect because it is cooked.*

10–12 thin Asparagus Stalks, cut into 3-in. segments

2 med. Red Bell Peppers, seeds and ribs removed, cut into matchsticks

2 med. Orange or Yellow Bell Peppers, seeds and ribs removed, cut into matchsticks

1/2 cup Snow Peas

1/4 cup Olive Oil

1 Yellow Onion, thinly sliced

1 Tbs. fresh grated Ginger

4 cloves minced Garlic

1 1/2 tsp. ground Cumin

1 Tbs. Curry Powder

1/2 tsp. Cinnamon

1/2 cup Pine Nuts

1 tsp. Real Salt™ or Bragg™ Liquid Aminos to taste

1/2 to 1 tsp. ground Mustard Seed

1/3 cup Coconut Milk (unsweetened)

1. Heat the olive oil in a large skillet or electric frypan over medium high heat. Add the asparagus and snow peas, and cook, stirring constantly, until they barely begin to brighten and soften. Add the onions and garlic, and reduce the heat to medium. Continue to cook until onions soften a bit. Add the bell peppers and steam-fry with a little water if necessary to barely soften the peppers.

2. Add the ginger, cumin, curry, cinnamon, and mustard seed, and a little more olive oil, and continue to stir-mix and cook. Add the salt, pine nuts and coconut milk, and cook until desired softness. I keep my veggies medium-crisp. Serve warm with the Autumn Curry Crepes, or can also be served over rice or any other cooked grain you prefer.

# Autumn Curry Crepes with Curried Veggie Filling

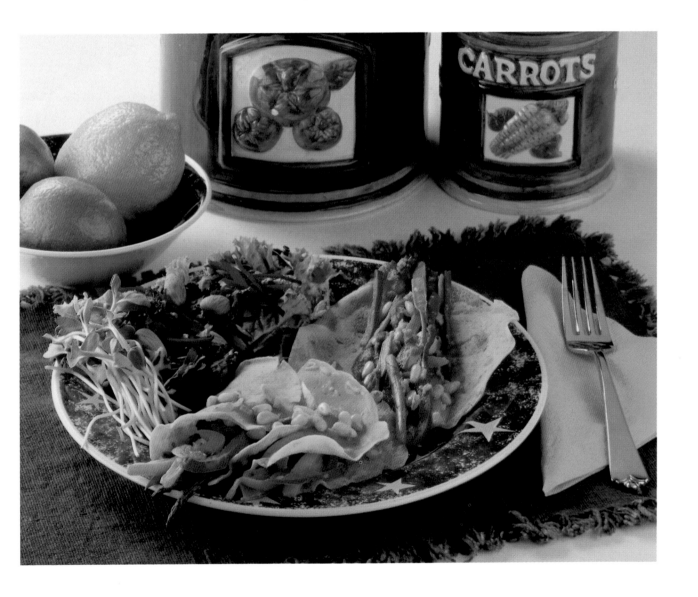

# Cold Tofu Pockets

1 pkg. firm or extra firm FRESH Tofu
3 Scallions
1/4 cup chopped fresh Coriander
1/4 Red Bell Pepper
1 tsp. Sesame Seeds
1 cup Bragg™ Liquid Aminos

Soak sesame seeds overnight. Drain tofu. Cut in half on the diagonal to form two triangles, then cut a pocket in each triangle. Finely chop the scallion, coriander, and pepper. Combine with sesame seeds. Stuff half the scallion mixture into each piece of tofu. Pour Liquid Aminos over tofu pockets and marinate in refrigerator for 10 minutes before serving.

# Vegetable Steam-Fry

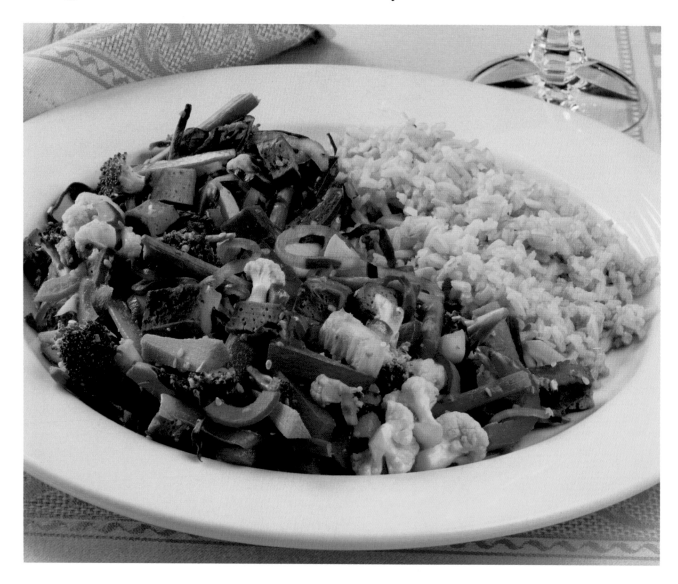

# Vegetable Steam-Fry

Heat up electric frypan. Add small amount of water and steam-fry the ginger and garlic for a couple of minutes. Pour in veggies and tofu and steam-fry until veggies are very bright and slightly softened. Pour the steam-fry sauce mixture over the top and steam for one or two more minutes. Serve immediately!

Variation: Sometimes I add pine nuts or sweet pecans to enrich this dish!

1–2 tsp. fresh grated Ginger (use a hand grater)
2–3 cloves Garlic, crushed
1/2 cup Broccoli (cut small)
1/2 cup Cauliflower, slices
1/2 cup Red Peppers, strips
1/2 cup Onion slices
1/2 cup Yellow Squash
1 cup Pea Pods
(Other veggies as desired, cut julienne)
1 cup fried Tofu (or use marinated tofu from the health food store)
1/4 tsp. Real Salt™

Steam-fry Sauce:
1/3 cup Water or Veggie Stock
1 tsp. Stir-Fry Ginger Spice (Spice Hunter)
Juice of half a Lemon or Lime
Bragg™ Liquid Aminos to taste

# Maren's Tortilla Pockets

*This makes 4 sealed pocket sandwiches and they are delicious! Serve with soup or salad.*

1. Buy a "Snack 'n Sandwich Maker" by White-Westinghouse ($17.00 at K-mart)
2. Use Alvarado Street Burrito size Sprouted Wheat Tortillas.
3. Make a 5"x 9" cardboard rectangle pattern.
4. Put heat setting on appliance at 3 or 4. Heat open.
5. Place your pattern in the middle of your stack of tortillas and cut a rectangle with a sharp knife. (Use remaining top and bottom pieces and make into chips by baking on a cookie sheet at 325° for 10 minutes.)
6. Place one tortilla rectangle on the bottom of appliance. Press down lightly with finger to find the center of the 4 triangles. Place fillings into each center of the triangles, keeping it away from the edges. Put another tortilla rectangle on top and close and lock lid for about 3 minutes, or until lightly golden.

Here are some filling suggestions:

• Hummus, pesto, salsa, Bragg's Aminos and alfalfa sprouts.
• Jasmine or basmati rice, black beans, salsa, Bragg's Aminos, Mexican Seasoning and avocado.
• Grated Vegetables, a squirt of olive oil, and Bragg's or Real Salt™.

# Sprouted Cereal

Soak grain overnight in distilled water. Drain and set jar on its side to sprout. Rinse sprouts morning and evening, and sprout for two days. Add enough water to sprouts to blend in blender. Pour into saucepan and cook until toasty warm. May be served in a bowl with soy milk.

2 cups Wheat or Rye Grains (organic, unstored)
1/2–1 tsp. Cinnamon

85

# Roasted Butternut/Celery Soup with Caramelized Onions

*This soup is a satisfying soup for chilly Autumn and Winter days. It is also delicious made with pumpkin and makes a great breakfast, lunch, dinner, or snack.*

2 Butternut Squash

3 Celery Stalks cut in big chunks

1 Onion, peeled and chopped in big chunks

1 Onion, peeled and sliced into thin rings for garnish

2 TB Olive or UDO's Oil

3-4 Cups Veggie Stock (I use Pacific Brand)

Cinnamon and Nutmeg or Salt and Pepper to taste.

1. Cut Squash in half and remove seeds. Lightly oil the cut side of the squash and chunks of celery and onion. Place squash cut side down and celery chunks on an oiled cookie sheet and roast in a 400 degree oven for about 45 minutes or until tender and lightly browned. Scoop out soft squash from the skins.

2. Puree the roasted vegetables in a blender or food processor with some of the stock. If you'd like a more smooth texture, pass the soup through a strainer into a clean pan. Add the rest of the stock and season to taste and keep warm.

3. To make the onion ring garnish, fry the onion in oil for 10 minutes until brown and somewhat crisp. Top soup and serve immediately.

# Veggie-Borscht

6 cups Veggie Broth

1 cup each Carrots (shredded), Beets (roughly chopped), Onions (thinly sliced)

1 1/2 cups Cabbage, shredded

1 Red Pepper (shredded)

Vegetized or Real Salt™ to taste

Pepper to taste

Combine broth, carrots, beets, and onion in large saucepan. Cook gently until becoming tender. Add cabbage and red pepper, salt and pepper to taste, and cook 5 minutes more. The soup will have a richer flavor if cooled completely before serving time, then reheated.

# Tofu Patties

*Serves 6.*

1 carton FRESH Tofu, drained

3 Tbs. Onion, chopped

3/8 tsp. Real Salt™

1 cup Zucchini, grated

1/2 Tbs. Vegetable Broth Mix

Egg Replacer equal to 2 eggs

Slice tofu and steam 5–10 minutes. Chop and drain well. Steam-fry onions. Add vegetable broth mix and zucchini and stir well. Add salt, tofu, and egg replacer and combine all ingredients. Make into patties. Put on sprayed baking sheets and flatten slightly. Bake lightly at 350°. Turn patties when bottoms are barely brown. Finish baking—do not overbake.

# Sprouted Bean Casserole

*Serves 6.*

Steam-fry the onion and garlic. Add leeks, Bragg™ Aminos, and pepper. Simmer 15 minutes. Add chopped pepper and simmer 5 minutes. Pour over beans in casserole dish. Stir gently. Bake at 350° for 15 minutes.

1 cup Mung Beans, sprouted
1 cup baby Lima Beans, sprouted
1 cup Pinto Beans, sprouted
1 large Onion, chopped
1 large Red or Green Pepper, finely chopped
1 clove Garlic, finely chopped
3 cups chopped Leeks
3 Tbs. Bragg™ Liquid Aminos
Freshly ground Pepper to taste

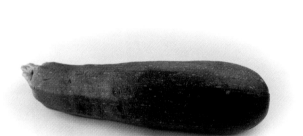

# Zucchini Italian Style

*Serves 8.*

1. Wash, trim ends, and slice zucchini. In a saucepan, steam-fry garlic, onion, and sliced zucchini over low heat, 10 minutes, turning and moving mixture occasionally.

2. Remove zucchini mixture from heat and sieve in tomatoes with pepper. Blend lightly and thoroughly. Turn mixture into a casserole dish, cover and simmer 30 minutes.

3. Add the olive oil to the dish before serving.

8–10 med. Zucchini
2/3 cup Onion, coarsely chopped
1 1/2 cups Tomatoes
1 tsp. Real Salt™
2 cloves Garlic, minced
1/8 tsp. Pepper
3 Tbs. Olive Oil

# Tofu Stew

*Serves 8.*

1. In a 3-quart pan with a lid, steam-fry the sliced onions. Add water, bay leaf, kale. Cover and simmer until kale begins to soften. Remove bay leaf. Add green beans and quartered onions, and continue to simmer until beans are tender.

2. Meanwhile, drain and slice tofu, and add to the pan to warm, or steam separately in steamer. Season if desired. Arrange tofu on top of stew to serve.

2 med. Onions, sliced
3 cups Water
1 Bay Leaf
3 Kale leaves, torn to bite-size
1 1/2 cups fresh Green Beans
2 Leeks, cut to bite-size
3 large Onions, quartered
1 pkg. FRESH Tofu, firmness of choice

# Ashley's Vegetable Nori Roll-Ups

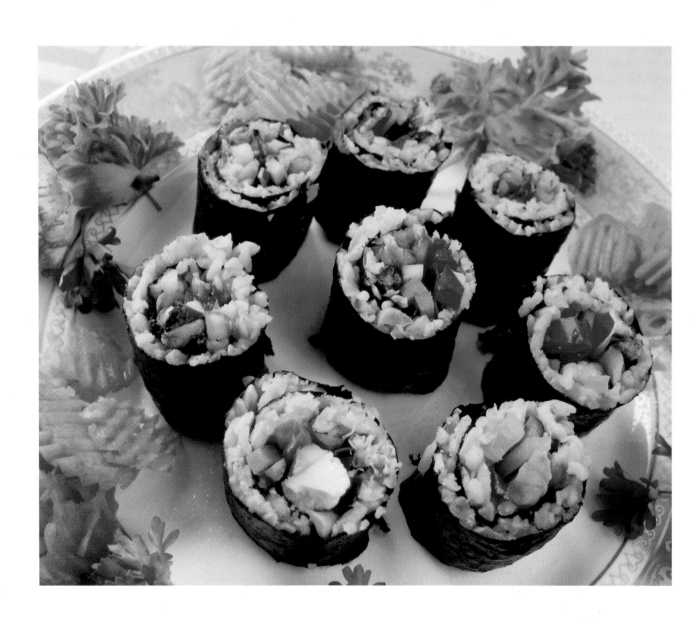

# Ashley's Vegetable Nori Roll-Ups

*Makes 2 to 3 rolls.*

1. In a small bowl, combine the lemon juice, Bragg™ Aminos, oil, and cinnamon or cayenne. Place the vegetables in a shallow pan and pour the lemon juice mixture over them.

2. Drain the vegetables thoroughly by tossing them in a colander or blotting them with paper towels.

3. Spread a thin layer of rice over each nori sheet, leaving about a 1/3-inch nori border at the end. Arrange the marinated vegetables on nori sheets; top them with a lot of sprouts and roll them up. Let sit until they will hold their form and cut into bite size pieces with a sharp knife.

Variations:
Use any vegetables and sprouts you like. Also serve with dips or sauces to go on top.

2 cups cooked Rice (basmati or brown)
1 pkg. Nori Sheets
Juice of 1 Lemon
2 Tbs. Bragg™ Liquid Aminos
1 tsp. Extra-Virgin Olive Oil or Flax Seed Oil
Dash of Cinnamon or Cayenne Pepper
2 Carrots, slivered
3 Scallions, slivered
1 Avocado, slivered
1 Zucchini, slivered
1 Cucumber, slivered
Alfalfa Sprouts
Buckwheat or Sunflower Seed Sprouts

# Stuffed Cabbage Rolls

*Serves 4.*

1. Grease a shallow, 2-quart range-top casserole with a tight-fitting lid. Remove and discard wilted outer leaves from cabbage. Rinse and cut in half through core. Remove eight large leaves. Shred enough remaining cabbage to yield 2 cups and spread into casserole dish. Add bay leaf, garlic clove, and set casserole aside. Pour boiling water into a large pan to 1-inch level. Add the eight leaves of cabbage and the salt. Cover and simmer 2–3 minutes.

2. Meanwhile, steam-fry chopped onion, tofu, pepper, and Liquid Aminos. Place one-quarter cup of this mixture into the center of each of the eight cabbage leaves, and roll each leaf, tucking ends in. Secure with wooden picks and place on shredded cabbage in a casserole dish.

3. Stir veggie broth mix into cold veggie broth, and pour over cabbage rolls with a few grains of pepper. Cover and simmer over low heat, 30 minutes. Remove bay leaf and picks and serve.

1 medium head of Cabbage
1 Bay Leaf
1 clove Garlic
1 cup Onion, finely chopped
1 pkg. drained FRESH Tofu (break into fine pieces)
1/8 tsp. Black Pepper
1/2 tsp. Real Salt™ or Vegetized Salt
1 tsp. Bragg™ Liquid Aminos
3 cups Vegetable Broth
1/2 cup Vegetable Broth Mix

# Curried Squash Dhal

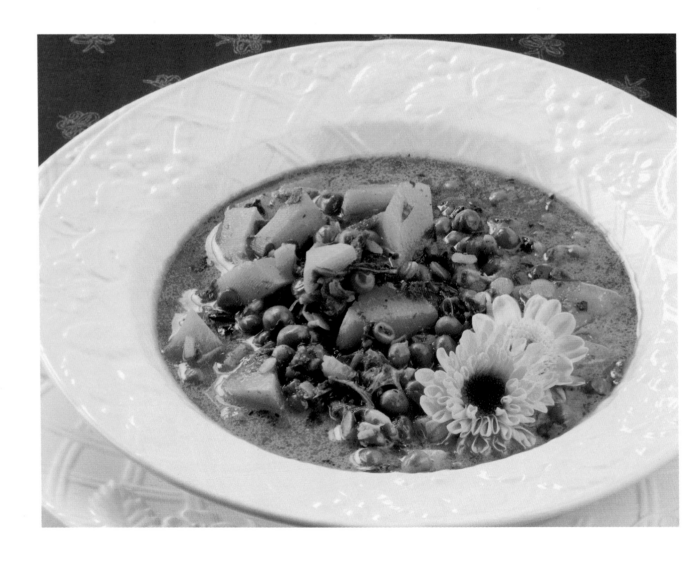

# Curried Squash Dhal

*You can use any kind of squash for this wonderfully warm dish. This can be made thick as a stew and served over rice, or thinned down as a soup that's great to start the day on a wintry morning!*

1. Combine onion, almond milk, garlic, chili peppers, ginger root, garam masala, sun-dried tomatoes, cumin, cinnamon, salt, turmeric, coriander, and 3 Tbs. stock or water in a blender. Purée mixture to a paste, scraping down the sides of the blender a few times.

2. Heat oil in a large saucepan, then add the spice paste and cook, stirring often, for 10 minutes. Add remaining stock, tomatoes, and butternut squash. Cook over medium heat, stirring often, until squash is just tender, about 20 minutes.

3. Mix in black-eyed beans, green peas, and spinach. Continue to cook, stirring often, until spinach is tender, about 10 more minutes. Remove from heat. Taste and adjust seasonings; stir in the mint just before serving. Yum!

1 med. Yellow Onion, quartered

1/2 can unsweetened Coconut or Almond Milk

3 cloves Garlic, sliced

2 Serrano or Thai Chili Peppers, seeded or diced

1 Tbs. fresh Ginger Root, minced

2 tsp. Garam Masala

1 tsp. ground Cumin

1/2 tsp. Cinnamon

1 tsp. Real Salt™

1/4 tsp. Turmeric

1/4 tsp. ground Coriander

2 cups Vegetable Stock or Water

1 Tbs. Udo's Choice® Oil or Olive Oil

2 cups fresh Tomatoes, diced

2–4 Sun-dried Tomatoes, minced

4 cups Butternut Squash, peeled and diced

2 cups Black-eyed Beans or Lentils, cooked

2 cups Spinach or Kale, chopped

1 cup Green Peas

3 Tbs. Mint, minced

# Zippy Garbanzo Spread

*Yield: 3 cups.*

Blend all in blender until smooth. Spread on sprouted whole wheat tortillas, topped with alfalfa sprouts, or eat with veggies.

4 cups sprouted, cooked Garbanzo Beans (Chickpeas)

3 Tbs. Tahini

3 Lemons or Limes

5–6 cloves of fresh Garlic, pressed

1 med. Onion, chopped

2 Tbs. dried Parsley

Dash of Cumin

1 tsp. Real Salt™

1 tsp. Coriander

Dash Cayenne or Chili Powder or Spice Hunter's "Zip"

1/4 cup Water

# Baked Falafel Fritters

*Makes 2 1/2 dozen. This recipe is wonderfully fast to whip up in your food processor. Fresh cilantro and the red hot chili pepper add fun color. (The red hot chili pepper is not that hot, but remember to take the ribs and seeds out of the middle first.) I serve these warm in cabbage leaves, rolled up as hors d'oeuvres, but they would also make a great side dish to a big salad or could even be thrown into a wrap or pita sandwich too! These are very hearty because they have both chickpeas and beans, making them high in calcium and protein. I use different kinds of beans to change the flavor and color of the fritters. The other plus is that they are baked instead of deep-fried like most falafel. Bon Appetit!*

8 oz. (1 cup) Beans, soaked overnight (drain well and cook in boiling water for about 10 minutes, or you could use canned in a pinch. I use black-eyed beans, cranberry beans, or lima beans.)

1/4 cup fresh Parsley, coarsely chopped

1/4 cup fresh Cilantro, coarsely chopped

1 1/2 cups canned Chickpeas, rinsed and drained (15 oz. can)

1 clove Garlic, minced

1 tsp. Cumin

1 tsp. Turmeric

1 Red Hot Chili Pepper, seeds and ribs removed, minced

1 Tbs. fresh Lime Juice

3 Tbs. Flour (spelt, millet, or whole wheat)

2 heads Butter Lettuce or Savoy Cabbage, leaves separated, tear big ones in half

6 cherry Tomatoes, quartered; or 1 small Tomato, finely chopped

Tahini Tofu Sauce (see recipe below)

1 Tbs. toasted or raw Sesame Seeds

1 tsp. Salt

1/4 cup Red Onion, chopped

1. In the bowl of a food processor, process the parsley and the cilantro until fine. Add the chickpeas, beans, garlic, cumin, turmeric, salt, 1/4 cup of the red onion, the chili pepper, and lime juice. Pulse until the mixture forms a very thick paste that is fairly smooth (this will involve scraping the sides down and processing a few times.) Add the flour, and pulse to combine. Transfer the mixture to a bowl and set aside. This mixture can be made one day ahead and refrigerated in an airtight container.

2. On a non-stick cookie sheet drop falafel mixture 1 Tbs. at a time and bake at 350° for 10–12 minutes. You can also brush these with olive oil and bake until golden brown if you like.

3. Serve each fritter warm on a piece of lettuce or cabbage cup. Garnish with the remaining onions, tomatoes, a dollop of Tahini Tofu Sauce, and a sprinkling of sesame seeds. Wrap up the cabbage around the fritter and eat like a finger food hors d'oeuvre, or serve by a salad for a great meal!

# Tahini Tofu Sauce

*Makes 2/3 cup. Serve this creamy, cool sauce with Baked Falafel Fritters, or use as a dip for fresh veggie stix or on top of steamed veggies. Can also be used as a main spread in a wrap!*

1 Garlic clove, finely chopped

2 Tbs. (or more) fresh Lemon or Lime Juice

1/4 cup Tahini

1 1/2 tsp. Bragg™ Liquid Aminos, or 1/2 to 1 tsp. Salt

1 Tbs. Olive Oil

1/3 cup soft silken Tofu (Nori brand)

Sesame Seeds, raw or toasted, for garnish

In the food processor, put the garlic, lemon juice, tahini and Bragg's. Process until combined. With the machine running, slowly add the olive oil through the feed tube, then add the soft tofu and pulse until smooth. Garnish with sesame seeds. This sauce can be stored in the refrigerator in an airtight container for a day or two.

To dry-toast sesame seeds, heat a heavy skillet over medium-low heat. Add the sesame seeds and shake the skillet gently to move the seeds around so that they toast evenly and do not burn. Toast the seeds until they are aromatic and barely take on color. Allow them to cool slightly before serving.

# Okra and Tomatoes Creole

Wash okra, cut off stem ends, slice and set aside. Chop onion and green pepper, steam-fry in a large skillet to transparent stage. Add okra and tomatoes. Stir in mixture of salt, pepper, curry powder, lecithin, and thyme. Simmer, covered, 30–40 minutes, or until okra is tender.

4 cups sliced Okra
1 cup chopped Onion
1/3 cup chopped Green Pepper
2 cups chopped Tomatoes
1/2 tsp. Real Salt™
1/8 tsp. Black Pepper
1/8 tsp. Curry Powder
1/8 tsp. Thyme
1 tsp. powdered Lecithin

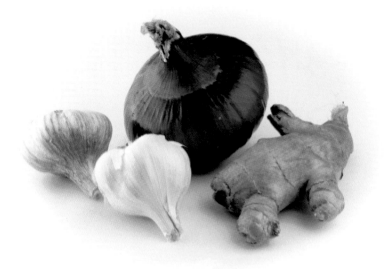

# Steam-Fried Sprouts

Steam-fry the onion and pepper in skillet, with Liquid Aminos. Add sprouts and steam gently for 30 seconds. Serve immediately.

2 Tbs. Bragg™ Liquid Aminos
1/2 cup finely chopped Onion
1/2 cup finely chopped Green or Red Pepper
2 cups fresh Bean Sprouts, any kind

# Refried Beans

Steam-fry onions and garlic. Purée pinto beans in food processor or blender. Pour puréed beans into the skillet. Stir beans constantly on low to medium heat until thickened; season while cooking. Serve hot with vegetables. Yield: 3 cups.

3 cups cooked Pinto Beans
1/2 cup Onion, chopped
1 tsp. minced Garlic
Garlic Powder to taste
Cayenne Pepper to taste
Black Pepper to taste

# Sunrise Asian Salad

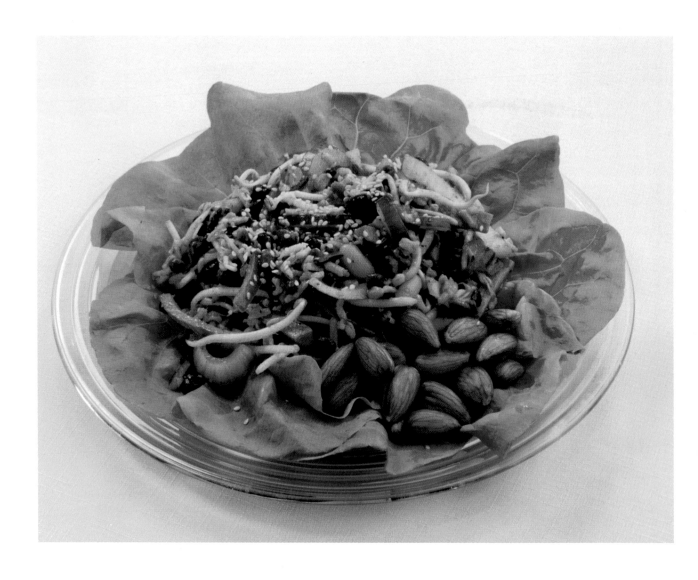

# Sunrise Asian Salad

*This is a hearty, chewy salad with the addition of beans and wild rice.*

1. Place beans and rice into large bowl.
2. In small food processor, place lemon juice, Bragg™ aminos, garlic, curry powder, ginger and pepper. Gradually add olive oil and process until well emulsified.
3. Pour dressing over bean/rice mixture. Add remaining vegetables. Toss well and then chill for 2 hours before serving.

1/2 cup Adzuki Beans
1/2 cup Black Beans
1/2 cup Black-Eyed Peas
1/2 cup Brown Rice
1/2 cup Wild Rice
1/2 med. Red Onion, sliced thinly
1/3 cup fresh Lemon Juice
1 Tbs. Bragg™ or 1 tsp. Real Salt™
1 tsp. Curry Powder
1 clove Fresh Garlic, minced
1 tsp. Zip or 2 tsp. Black Pepper
1 inch cubed of fresh Ginger, grated
2/3 cup Olive Oil
1 Carrot, julienned (use mandoline)
1/2 cup Snowpeas, trimmed and sliced
1 cup Bean Sprouts or 1 cup Sprouts, any kind (I use Pro-Vita mix sprouts from Life Sprouts)

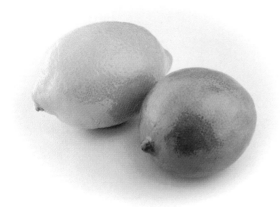

# Tofu Spinach Quiche

Pastry:
1. Combine the ingredients, and knead the dough into a cohesive ball.
2. Roll out the pastry on a floured board and press it into a greased pie dish.

Filling:
1. Sauté the onions in oil until they are transparent.
2. Add the dill weed, parsley, spinach (defrosted), and salt and mix them in well.
3. Blend the tofu in a processor with the soy milk if it is difficult to blend on its own. (You might also put the parsley into the blender to chop it up more easily.)
4. Pour this over the vegetable mixture and mix it thoroughly.
5. Place the filling in the pastry case and bake it at 375° for about 30 minutes.

Pastry:
4 cups Whole Wheat Flour
6 Tbs. Vegetable Oil
Pinch of Real Salt™
A little cold Water

Filling:
2 Onions (diced)
3/4 cup Vegetable Oil
2 Tbs. Parsley (chopped)
2 Tbs. Dill Weed
2 cups Spinach (chopped & cooked)
2 (10 oz.) packets frozen Spinach
Real Salt™ to taste
2 cups Tofu
1/4 cup Soy Milk (if necessary)

# Nutty Mock Meat Loaf

1 cup Almonds, raw
2/3 cup Sunflower Seeds, raw
1/2 cup Brazil Nuts, raw
1/4 cup Flax Seed, ground
1/2 cup Water
2 small Onions, diced
1/2 cup Parsley, fresh
1/2 tsp. Real Salt™
1/2 tsp. Sweet Basil
1/2 tsp. Sage
1/3 tsp. Thyme

Sauce:
1/2 cup Almonds, ground
2 cups Water
1 tsp. Seasoning, your choice
2 Tbs. Arrowroot Flour
Dash of Cayenne Pepper
2 Tbs. Olive oil
1/4 tsp. Real Salt™

Preheat oven at 350°. Grind nuts and seeds in a processor, blender or grinder. Combine remaining dry ingredients, mix well. Add the water and mix again. Place in a well-oiled loaf pan and bake for 25 minutes at 350°.

Sauce:
Combine all ingredients, bring to a low boil and stir constantly. Turn heat down and simmer on low heat until thick. Pour over top of nut loaf.

Serve with tossed salad or steamed vegetables. This is a good snack and freezes well. As an option to the listed spices, I use Spice Hunter's Cowboy Barbecue Rub and 3 sun-dried tomatoes.

# Alexandra's Favorite Pasta

*Yield: 6 servings.*

2 tsp. Olive Oil
1 28 oz. can Plum Tomatoes, undrained
2 cloves Garlic, minced
16 oz. Spaghetti or Fettuccine, uncooked
8 oz. Almond Cheese
1/8 tsp. Red Pepper Flakes

1. Cube tomatoes, heat with juice over medium heat with garlic and olive oil for 20 minutes.
2. Meanwhile, cook pasta, drain, and place in serving bowl.
3. Add tomatoes, cheese, and red pepper flakes, toss.
4. Cover bowl for 5 minutes to allow cheese to melt.
5. Toss again before serving.

# Nutty Mock Meat Loaf

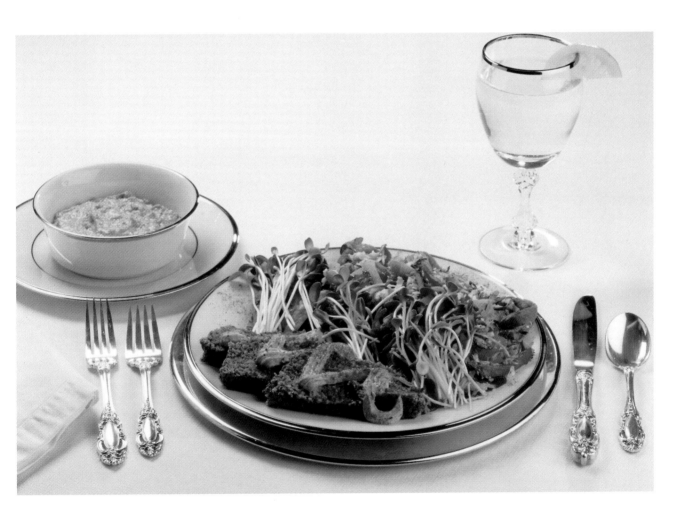

# Yummus Hummus

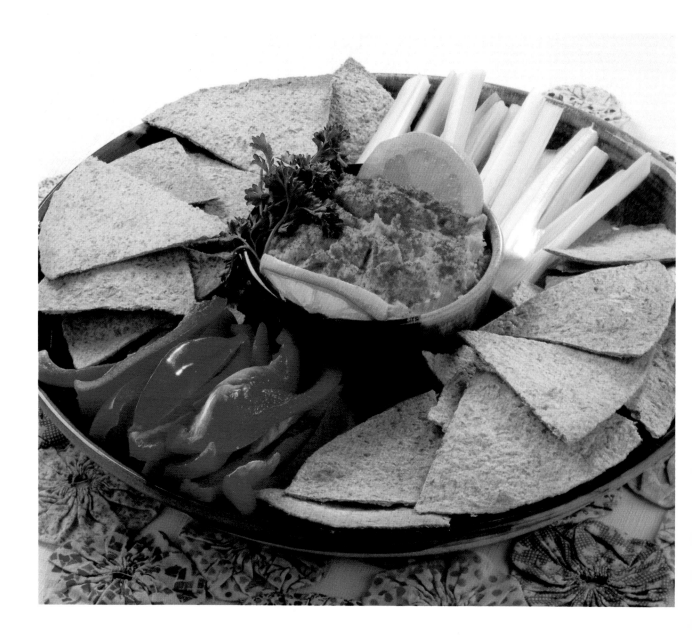

# Green Mayonnaise

1 lb. Tofu, drained
2 Avocados
1/2 Tbs. Curry Powder
3 Tbs. Lemon Juice
Salt to taste
"Zip" to taste

Guacamole:
1 Tomato, chopped, peeled
1/2 Onion, chopped, peeled
2–3 seeded Green Chili Peppers

Blend in a processor until mayonnaise consisistency.

To make Guacamole from the Green Mayonnaise recipe, add the ingredients listed under "Guacamole" to the Green Mayonnaise.

Variation: add parsley, chives, tarragon, or other spices of choice.

# Yummus Hummus

2–3 Tbs. Olive Oil
Juice of 1 lemon
1–2 garlic cloves minced
1/8–1/4 cup Tahini (raw)
1 17-oz. jar Garbanzo Beans, drained (save water from beans)
Real Salt™ to taste
1/2–1 tsp. Garlic Herb Bread Seasoning (Spice Hunter)
1/2–1 tsp. Cumin
"Zip" to taste

1. In a food processor put oil, lemon juice, garlic and tahini and process until smooth.

2. Add beans and seasonings and process until creamy.

3. You may need to thin with extra water (from beans) to desired consistency. Serve on wraps, with raw veggies or in pita sandwiches.

# Almond/Carrot/Ginger-Stuffed Zucchini

1 large Onion, peeled and chopped
2 Tbs. Olive Oil
4 medium Zucchini
1 clove Garlic, minced
4 medium Carrots, scraped and finely diced
1 tsp. grated fresh Ginger
2/3 cup soaked Almonds, chopped, or raw unsoaked Macadamia Nuts, chopped
Real Salt ® to taste
"Zip" or Pepper to taste

1. Preheat oven to 375°.
2. Sauté onion in the oil in a medium saucepan for 5 minutes. Half the zucchini lengthwise and scoop out the soft centers to make good cavities for stuffing.
3. Chop the scooped-out zucchini and add it to the onion along with the garlic, carrot and ginger. Cover and sauté gently for about 10 minutes, until the veggies are slightly soft.
4. Remove from heat and add the chopped almonds or macadamias and seasonings to taste.
5. Place the zucchini skins in an oiled shallow casserole and fill them with the carrot mixture. Cover and bake for about 30–40 minutes. Serve immediately.

# Edamame Patties

*These are a hardy little veggie burger that can be pan fried if you're in a hurry, or dehydrated for 4-6 hours to make a more crusty outside. They are made with a base of Edamame (Soy Beans from Pods) that you can find in your health food store in the frozen section.*

3 Tbs. Flax seeds, ground into powder (using blender or coffee grinder)

6 Tbs. Water

10-oz. pkg. Vegetable Soy Beans (Sno Pack carries a brand already de-podded or you can get them in the pod and slip the beans out yourself.)

1 Carrot, grated fine or processed to fine pulp

2 cloves Garlic

1 tsp. Dried Onion

1/2 cup Parsley

1/2 tsp. Dried Mustard

1/2 tsp. Turmeric

1 tsp. Mexican seasoning (Spice Hunter)

1/3 tsp. Deliciously Dill (Spice Hunter)

1 tsp. Real Salt™

2 Sun-dried Tomatoes (packed in Olive Oil)

Grind flax seeds to powder put in a bowl. Add the water and stir to mix well. Set aside to gel up.

Put carrot, garlic, dried onion, sundried tomatoes, flax mixture, and all spices into a food processor and process to desired consistency. (I do this quite smooth.) Then add the edamame beans and process until well mixed. You can make them coarse and more chunky with the beans showing or smoother and more mixed if you like. Also you can use more edamame beans if the mixture seems to be too moist. They should be able to form into a patty easily. Then make into small patties and put into a dehydrator for 4–6 hours, or use a little grape seed oil and dip the patties in some sprouted wheat tortilla crumbs and fry on both sides. Serve with the Rich Raw Tomato Sauce on top for a real treat!

*Optional:* You can use all sorts of different spices for these. Sometimes I use Italian Pizza seasonings, or Garlic Herb Bread Seasonings by Spice Hunter. Also you could add some garbanzo or other beans of choice to stretch the recipe or add more bean flavors. Experiment! Enjoy!

# Thick Purée of White Bean Soup

*Serves 8.*

2 lb. dried White Beans, washed and picked over

2 Onions, chopped

3 large cloves Garlic, minced

7 cups Water

1 Bay Leaf

2 sprigs Parsley

1 whole leaf Swiss Chard, sliced crosswise

Real Salt™ or Bragg™ Liquid Aminos

Black Pepper, freshly ground

Soak beans 24 hours, in three times their volume of pure water, and drain. Steam-fry onions and one clove garlic until onions are tender. Put in large pot with 7 cups water, add drained beans, remaining garlic, bay leaf, parsley, and chard, and bring to a boil. Reduce heat, cover, and simmer 1 hour. Add salt and continue to simmer until beans are tender. Remove bay leaf and parsley. Purée soup in batches in a blender. Return to pot and adjust seasonings. This can be frozen.

# Hearty Harvest Casserole

*Serves 12.*

Steam-fry onion and green peppers. Combine all ingredients in a casserole dish. Cover. Bake at 350° for 1 hour. Barley should be tender.

2 large Onions, cut and separated into rings 3/4" thick

1 each med. Green and Red Pepper, cut into 1" strips

1 cup sprouted Barley, partially cooked (save 1 cup water)

1 cup Barley Water (saved above)

4 Tbs. Vegetable Broth mix

3 med. Carrots, cut into chunks

2 large Tomatoes, peeled and quartered

2 med. Zucchini cut into 1 1/2-inch chucks

1 lb. Green Beans, snapped in half

1/2 head Cauliflower florets

2 cloves Garlic, crushed

1 Tbs. Real Salt™

1/4 tsp. Black Pepper, 1 tsp. Paprika

1/4 cup Parsley, chopped

*Hearty Harvest Casserole*

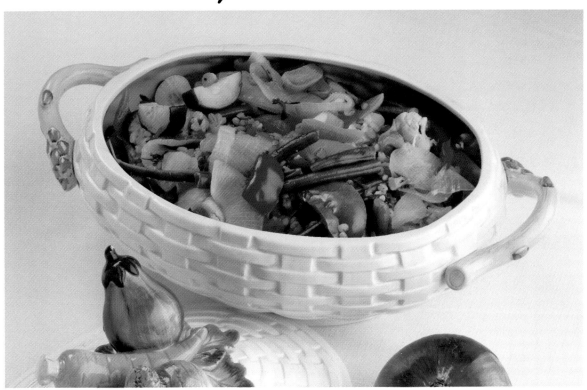

# Italian Tomato Sauce

*Yield: 14 servings. Per serving 1/2 cup.*

2 28-oz. cans Italian Tomatoes (crushed)
1 tsp. Basil
1/2 tsp. Oregano
1 6-oz. can Tomato Paste
1 Bay Leaf
5 tsp. Garlic (minced)
1/2 tsp. Cayenne Pepper

1. Mix all ingredients; simmer on stove for 2 hours. Use in your favorite Italian recipe or serve over spaghetti.

# Green Beans Lyonnaise Style

1 lb. Green Beans
1/2 cup boiling Water
1/2 tsp. Real Salt™
1 cup thinly sliced Onion
1/4 tsp. Black Pepper
1/4 tsp. Nutmeg
3 tsp. Flax Seed Oil
1 Tbs. Parsley

Wash green beans, break off ends, then cut lengthwise into fine strips. Carefully place beans and salt into saucepan of boiling water. Cook, loosely covered, until tender-crisp. Meanwhile, in skillet steam-fry the onion. Drain beans and add to skillet with a mixture of salt, pepper, and nutmeg. Sauté 5 minutes. Add flax seed oil and parsley. Toss well and serve.

## Green Beans Lyonnaise Style

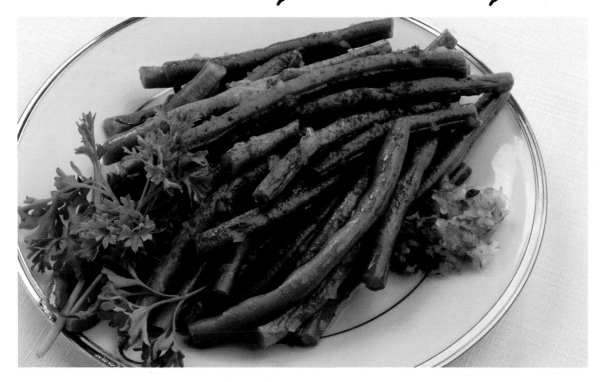

# CHAPTER 6

# *Roof*

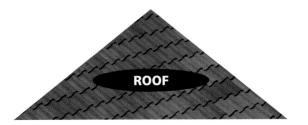

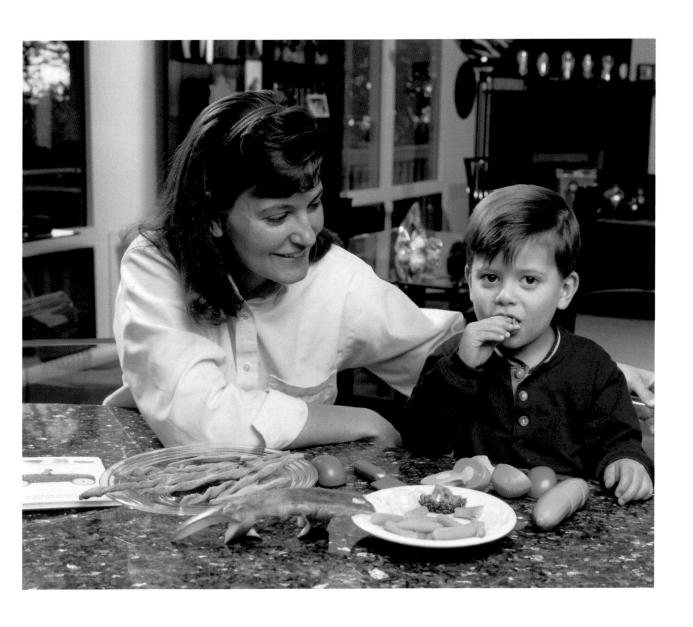

*When a proper diet is not present, medicine is of no use.*
*When a proper diet is present, medicine is of no need.*

—Deepak Chopra

## House of Health Snack Food Recipes

Welcome to the House of Healthy Snacks! Here are Roof recipes to top off your healthy alkalizing diet and lifestyle.

So you've noticed that I don't have a dessert section in this recipe book. When we think of a dessert, we usually think of sweets, something sugary, starchy, and fattening, all of which would be acidic to the body. For this reason we really don't promote dessert, especially on top of a big meal, because the sugary dessert will basically sugar up the whole meal and cause excess fermentation, excess acid and gas during digestion. If you decide to indulge, eat dessert before your meal, or by itself, in between meals. The following healthy snacks could be used as dessert, or during sugar cravings, or when transitioning to better snack choices that lean towards alkaline.

Some of these Roof recipes travel really well, and make it possible for you to continually nourish yourself the best way possible. They satisfy the need for crunch and munch that kids of all ages need. So go ahead—snack for good health!

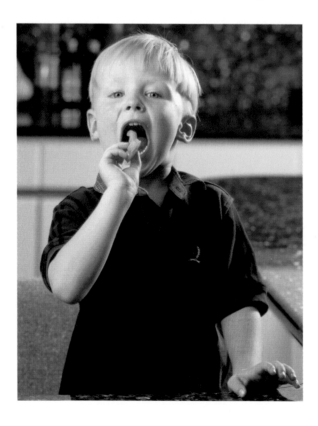
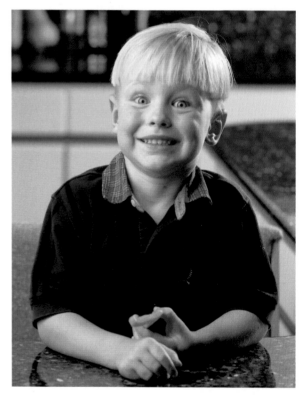

# Tofu/Avocado Dip

In a blender or food processor, combine tofu, lemon juice, garlic powder, onion, cilantro, and chili powder until well blended. Put the mixture in a bowl, add tomato and avocado and mix well. Chill and serve with chips or fresh veggies or put all ingredients in food processor. Process until smooth, serve chilled.

1 package soft FRESH tofu, drained
1 1/2 tsp. Lemon Juice
1 tsp. Garlic Powder
1 Tbs. diced Onion
2 Tbs. chopped fresh Cilantro
1/2 tsp. Chili Powder
1 small Tomato, diced (optional) or 2–3 Sun-dried Tomatoes
1 med. Avocado, mashed
1/2–1 tsp. Real Salt™

# Dried Veggies and Nuts for Crunch and Munch

*Dehydrated vegetables are great snacks and also come in handy to garnish your meals.*
*For veggies like onions, bell peppers and tomatoes, you can just slice and dehydrate until crisp.*
*These are also very pretty sprinkled over soups*

For root vegetables like hard squashes, carrots, yams, slice thinly and marinate in Bragg™ Liquid Aminos, garlic, ginger, and any spices you like. Marinate them up to an hour. Drain, and then dehydrate them until desired dryness or crispness. These are great with dips and patés too.

When dehydrating nuts, begin with soaked nuts and marinate in a shallow bowl with Bragg™ Liquid Aminos, garlic, ginger, and any spices you prefer. These can be marinated for 1 to 12 hours. Drain the nuts well, and place them in a dehydrator and dry until crunchy. Store in an airtight container in the fridge.

# Tahini (Sesame Seed Butter)

Combine in food processor or blender. Blend into a smooth paste. This is a protein food, for use with non-starchy vegetables. Use up quickly. Keep refrigerated, tightly covered.

1 cup Sesame Seeds
2 tsp. Flax Seed Oil

# Great Olé Guacamole

*The Mexican Seasoning and "Zip" really give this guacamole a kick! Use this as a dip for fresh veggies. Cut the veggies like bell peppers and cabbage with small cookie cutters for children.*

**Juice of 1 Lemon or Lime (or use both)**
**1 large Tomato**
**3 Avocados**
**1 tsp. Mexican Seasoning (Spice Hunter)**
**1/4 tsp. Cumin**
**1/2 tsp. "Zip"**

In a food processor fitted with an S-blade, blend the lemon juice with half the tomato and half the avocado until smooth. Finely dice the remaining half tomato. Mash the remaining avocado, leaving the pulp chunky. Combine both mixtures, seasoning with the Mexican Seasoning, cumin, "Zip," and additional lemon juice to taste, if desired. Olé!

# Avocado/Tomato Snack

**2 Avocados**
**1 small Eggplant, diced**
**3/4 Tbs. Curry Powder**
**2 Tbs. Lemon Juice**
**2 seeded Green Chili Peppers**
**Real Salt™ and seasoning to taste**
**2 or 3 Tomatoes, thickly sliced**

Blend all except tomatoes in blender until smooth. Spoon onto warmed tomato slices.

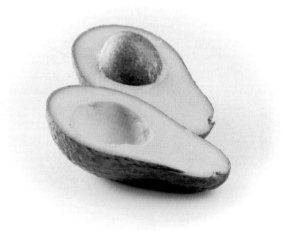

# Sweet Pepper Consommé

*Serves 6.*

**3 med. Red Peppers**
**2 Tomatoes**
**1 med. Onion**
**3/4 tsp. Real Salt™**
**1 whole clove Garlic**
**2 qt. boiling Water**

Cut the peppers in quarters, remove seeds. Quarter tomatoes and onion. Put all ingredients in boiling water. Simmer, covered, for one and a half hours. Strain and taste for seasoning. A delicate and delicious broth, which may be served hot or cold.

# Great Olé Guacamole

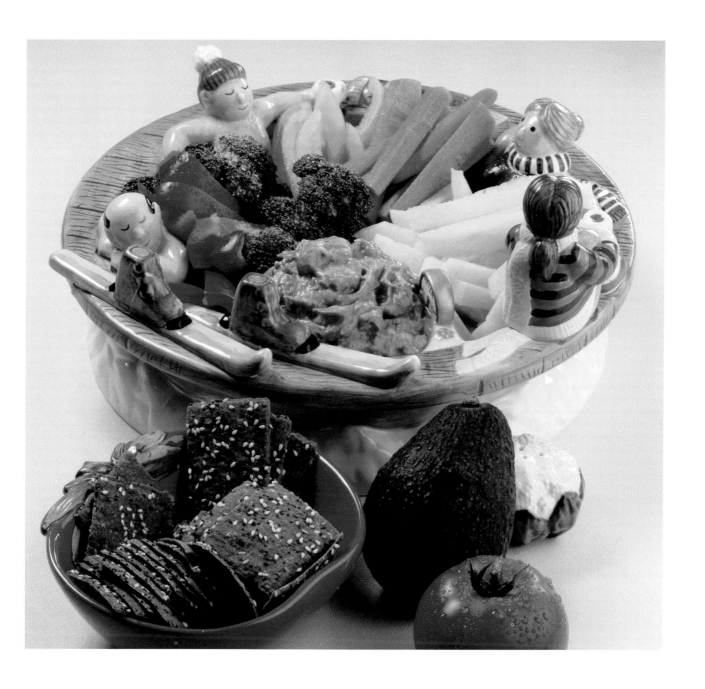

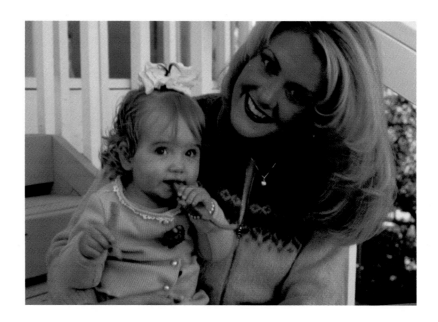

# Veggie Crunch Stix and Crackers

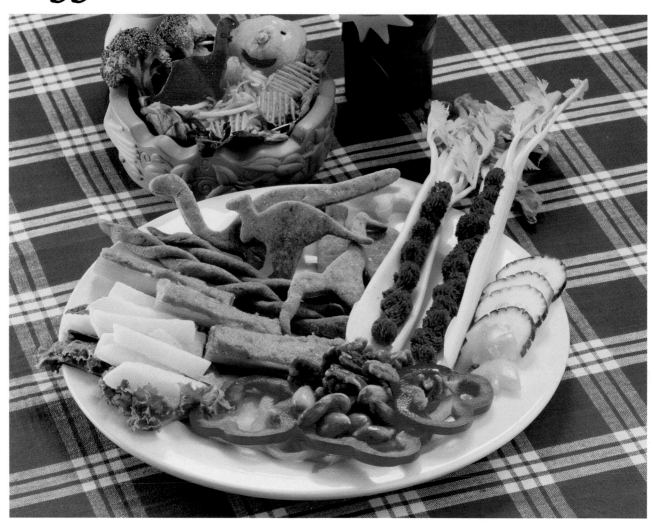

# Veggie Crunch Stix and Crackers

*These colorful snacks are a great way to wean children and adults from yeast breads. They are a wonderful grab-snack and also complement and give crunch to a vegan-based meal like soup and salad. They work up very fast and travel well. I use the small cookie cutters and make little dinosaurs, airplanes, and heart crackers. Also, you can season them any way you want by adding a couple of teaspoons of your favorite spice.*

1. In a food processor, pulse the flour, the salt, and baking powder to combine. Add the tofu and olive oil and pulse until the mixture resembles coarse meal. With the machine running, gradually add between 1/2–3/4 cup ice water or fresh veggie juice until the dough comes together in a soft ball (approx. 1 minute).

2. Turn the dough out onto a lightly floured surface. Form the dough into a smooth rectangle, about 4 x 6 inches, then roll out the dough into an 8 x 10-inch sheet, 1/4-inch thick. With a sharp knife cut the dough lengthwise into 1/4-inch-wide strips.

3. Using your hands, gently roll each strip into 16-inch long sticks. For a twisted version, grab each end of the dough strip with your fingers and carefully stretch and twist the strip in opposite directions. For crackers use cookie cutters (children love these!) and arrange on baking sheet. Arrange the sticks on two baking sheets, side by side but not touching, and press ends into the baking sheet to keep the sticks straight while they cook. If desired, brush each stick lightly with olive oil and sprinkle with salt or seasonings of your choice. Bake at 350° until firm and cooked through, 14–18 minutes.

4. Transfer the sticks or crackers to a wire rack to cool. Store in an airtight container at room temperature for two to three days.

**2 cups Spelt Flour (or other flours: all-purpose, millet, etc.)**
**1/2 to 1 tsp. Salt**
**1 1/2 tsp. Baking Powder**
**3 heaping Tbs. soft Tofu (Nori brand is good)**
**2 Tbs. Olive Oil**
**1–2 tsp. Seasonings of your choice (optional)**
**1/2–3/4 cup cold Water or fresh Vegetable Juice, or mix**

Variations:

*Beet Stix*
2 Tbs. Beet Juice, from 1 small beet. Combine with 1/2 cup cold water.

*Popeye Stix*
1/2 cup Parsley or Spinach Juice. Combine with 1/4 cup cold water.

*Bugs Bunny Stix*
1/4 cup Carrot Juice, from about 3 carrots. Combine with 1/4 cup cold water.

*Tomato Stix*
1/4 cup fresh Tomato Juice, with 1–2 Tbs. sun-dried tomato pesto. Combine with 1/3 cup cold water.

Spicing Variations:

*Curry/Turmeric Stix*
1 tsp. Curry Powder, with 1/2 tsp. ground Turmeric

*Cumin Stix*
2 tsp. ground Cumin

*Garlic Stix*
2 tsp. Garlic Herb Bread Seasoning (Spice Hunter)

*Mexi Stix*
2 tsp. Mexican Seasoning (Spice Hunter)

As always… Experiment!! and try different combinations.

# Crispy Buckwheat Groats

2 cups hulled Buckwheat Groats, soaked 6–8 hours

Bragg™ Liquid Aminos to taste

Lemon or Lime juice (I use both)

The Zip (Spice Hunter) or any seasoning to taste

Drain the buckwheat groats and put in a shallow bowl. Add Liquid Aminos and juice to cover. Add spices to taste. Soak in this solution for 1 hour, then drain again. Put groats in food dehydrator on teflex liners and dehydrate until dry (2–3 hours).

These are great little munchy snacks and can be used as croutons in a salad or wrap.

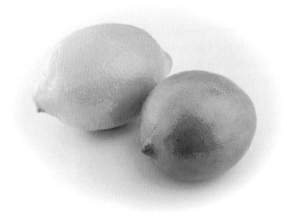

# Chilled Cucumber Refresher

*Serves 6.*

4 cups yeast-free Vegetable Broth

1 cup Cucumber, shredded

Dill Weed

Combine broth and cucumber, chill. Sprinkle each serving with dill weed.

# Zippy Cilantro Dip

1 or 2 hot Chili Peppers

1/2 cup chopped fresh Cilantro

2 cups frozen petite Peas, thawed

1 pkg. FRESH Tofu, drained

1 Tbs. Lemon Juice

1 tsp. ground Cumin

1/4 tsp. freshly ground Pepper

Real Salt™ to taste

1 med. Cucumber

Combine one-quarter of the cilantro and all other ingredients in a food processor until smooth, blending approximately 30 seconds on high. Refrigerate 1 hour. Lay overlapping thin cucumber slices and rim with the remaining cilantro. Serve with raw vegetables.

## Dehydrated Flax Chips

Soak the flax seeds in 2 cups water for 2 to 4 hours. Process the tomato, bell pepper, beet, garlic, Mexican spices, onion, and real salt. Keep it chunky. Add the soaked flax seeds into the blended mixture, and spoon 2-inch rounds onto a teflex sheet and dehydrate at 105°–110° for 8–12 hours, or to the desired crispness. Turn the crisps over after 4–6 hours to ensure even drying.

Optinal: Sprinkle sesame or soaked pumpkin seeds on top before dehydrating.

1 cup Flax Seeds

1 Tomato

1/2 Red Bell Pepper

1 clove Garlic

1–2 tsp. Mexican Seasoning, Italian, Garlic Herb Bread, or any other spice combo you like (Spice Hunter)

1/2 small Red Onion, or 1 tsp. dried Onion Flakes

1/2 Beet

Real Salt™ to taste

# *Dehydrated Flax Chips*

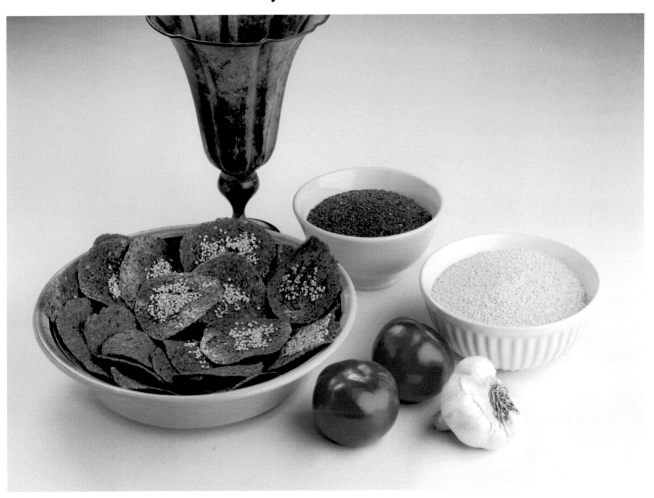

# Camper's Bread

2 cups Sprouted Wheat Flour
4 Tbs. non-aluminum Baking Powder
1 Tbs. Real Salt™
2 Tbs. Oil (Olive or Udo's Choice®)
1 cup pure Water

Mix dry ingredients, cut in oil, add water, and mix well. Grease frying pan, pour in batter, bake very slowly. Turn.

# Mock Pumpkin Pie

*This recipe was the result of trying to come up with something healthy in place of pumpkin pie at Thanksgiving. It is a healthy alternative made out of carrots. Experiment using pumpkin and other squashes.*

**Pie Crust**
2 cups raw Almonds
2–3 Tbs. Soy Milk or Almond Milk
2 Tbs. Wheat Bran Flakes

Place raw almonds in food processor and pulse-chop until fine. Add soy milk and bran one tablespoon at a time until mixture holds together. Press into pie plate evenly.

**Pie Filling**
1 lbs. Carrots, peeled and grated
1/2 tsp. Nutmeg
1/2 tsp. Cinnamon
1/8 tsp. Clove
1 tsp. Vanilla
1/2 cup Slivered Almonds, for garnish

Steam carrots until soft. Place in blender or food processor and process until smooth. Add spices and vanilla to taste. Pour mixture into almond crust. Garnish top of pie with slivered or whole almonds. Chill in fridge overnight and serve cold.

# Essene Bread

To each quart of sprouted grain, add 2/3 cup pure water. Grind up in a Vita-Mix®. Form into a small loaf and bake at 275° for 3 hours or until crust forms. Very moist.

# Leprechaun Surprise Dip

2 cups Spinach, very finely chopped
2 cups Parsley, very finely chopped
1 cup Green Onions, very finely chopped
1/2 cup Mock Mayo (see p. 62)

Mix well. Serve with fresh vegetables.

# Hearty Nut Filling

Mix all ingredients, can put in food processor if desired. Excellent to stuff celery sticks or with vegetables.

1/2 cup Almond Butter
1/4 cup finely chopped Green Pepper
1/4 cup grated Carrot
1 tsp. minced Onion
4 Tbs. Mock Mayo (see page 62)
1 1/2 tsp. Salt
1/2 med. Red Onion, finely chopped

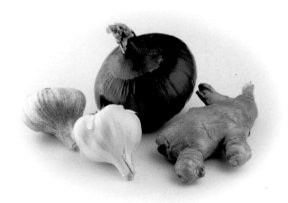

# Raw Pecan Paté

*This paté spreads well on tortillas and celery. The fresh raw pecans and shredded veggies make it a sweet paté that's great for children!*

In a food processor fitted with an S-blade, blend the pecans, onions, poultry spice, and basil leaves. Thin with enough water (optional) to desired consistency like paté. Add the grated veggies and poultry seasoning into the processor and keep blending until well mixed and moist. Stir in the minced parsley and mix well.

You can even make this into patties and warm in a food dehydrator to the desired warmth and crispness (4 to 8 hours) if you wish; or if you are in a hurry, you could warm the paté lightly in an electric skillet right before you serve it. Other spices can be added to the paté too, e.g., Spice Hunter's Vegetable Rub, Garlic Herb Bread Seasoning, California Pizza, or Cowboy Barbecue Rub. Experiment!

2 cups fresh raw Pecans
1/4–1/2 Red Onion
1–2 tsp. Poultry Spice (e.g., Spice Hunter)
4–6 fresh Basil Leaves
1/4 cup finely grated Carrots, Beets, and/or raw Squash
1/4 cup finely minced Parsley (optional)

# Almond Paté

In food processor, process the almonds, lemon juice, Liquid Aminos, and garlic until smooth. Store in an airtight container in the fridge.

Variations: This is a basic paté spread recipe. You can vary it by using pine nuts, sesame seeds, or other nuts like soaked hazelnuts or pecans. You can cream it up more by adding tahini. Also try to season it differently with various Spice Hunter spices. Fresh herbs or dehydrated veggies can color and flavor it up. Be daring and creative! Use to stuff peppers or celery. Spread on crackers or wraps.

3 cups soaked Almonds
1 cup Lemon Juice
1/4 cup Bragg™ Liquid Aminos
1/2–1 clove Garlic (could use roasted garlic too)

# Sprouted Wheat Bread

Sprout 2 cups wheat for two days, then grind. Make a pad 1/8-inch thick from this dough. Bake on a flat stone in full summer sun from morning until noon on one side, from noon until evening on the other side. If weather is bad, bake it in a slow oven until slightly crisp. This recipe is adapted from the Dead Sea Scrolls and is the same type of bread Jesus broke at the Last Supper. This is a tasty, hardtack-like bread.

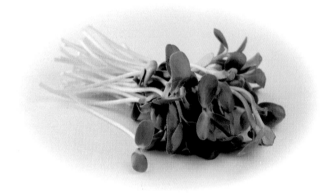

# Tofu Paté

1 lb. firm FRESH Tofu, drained
1 Tbs. Bragg™ Liquid Aminos
1 Tbs. Sesame Tahini
1 Tbs. Flax Seed Oil
2 Tbs. yeast-free Vegetable Broth
1 Tbs. minced Chives
1 Tbs. minced fresh Basil

Place all ingredients in a mixing bowl and mix thoroughly until smooth. Press the mixture into a mold and refrigerate for two hours.

Slice or scoop out and serve with non-starchy vegetables.

# Tomato Sauce

*Makes about 3 1/2 cups.*

1/2 cup Onion, chopped
1/2 cup Vegetable Stock
3 cups Tomatoes, coarsely chopped
1/2 tsp. each Oregano, Thyme, and Basil
1 tsp. Garlic Powder
Freshly ground Pepper

Cook onion in stock until soft. Add remaining ingredients. Bring to a boil, cover and simmer 30–45 minutes. Add other herbs and spices to flavor as desired. Store in a glass jar and refrigerate until ready to use. For good food combination, eat with celery, bell peppers, cucumbers, eggplant, okra, or summer squash.

# *Appendix A: Nutritional Charts*

# Table 1
# Food "Ash" pH

*The following is a list of common foods with an approximate, relative potential of acidity (-) or alkalinity (+), as present in one ounce of food.*

## Foods You Can Eat Freely

### Vegetables

| | |
|---|---|
| Brussels sprouts | +0.5 |
| Peas, ripe | +0.5 |
| Asparagus | +1.1 |
| Artichokes | +1.3 |
| Comfrey | +1.5 |
| Green cabbage, March harvest | +2.0 |
| Lettuce | +2.2 |
| Onion | +3.0 |
| Cauliflower | +3.1 |
| White cabbage | +3.3 |
| Green cabbage, December harvest | +4.0 |
| Savoy cabbage | +4.5 |
| Lamb's lettuce | +4.8 |
| Peas, fresh | +5.1 |
| Zucchini | +5.7 |
| Red cabbage | +6.3 |
| Rhubarb stalks | +6.3 |
| Leeks (bulbs) | +7.2 |
| Watercress | +7.7 |
| Spinach, March harvest | +8.0 |
| Chives | +8.3 |
| French cut beans (green beans) | +11.2 |
| Sorrel | +11.5 |
| Spinach (other than March) | +13.1 |
| Garlic | +13.2 |
| Celery | +13.3 |
| Cabbage lettuce, fresh | +14.1 |
| Endive, fresh | +14.5 |
| Cayenne pepper | +18.8 |
| Straw grass | +21.4 |
| Shave grass | +21.7 |
| Dog grass | +22.6 |
| Dandelion | +22.7 |
| Kamut grass | +27.6 |
| Barley grass | +28.7 |
| Soy sprouts | +29.5 |
| Sprouted radish seeds | +28.4 |
| Sprouted chia seeds | +28.5 |
| Alfalfa grass | +29.3 |
| Cucumber, fresh | +31.5 |
| Wheat Grass | +33.8 |

### Root Vegetables

| | |
|---|---|
| White radish (spring) | +3.1 |
| Rutabaga | +3.1 |
| Kohlrabi | +5.1 |
| Horseradish | +6.8 |
| Turnip | +8.0 |
| Carrot | +9.5 |
| Fresh red beet | +11.3 |
| Red radish | +16.7 |
| Summer black radish | +39.4 |

### Fruits

| | |
|---|---|
| Limes | +8.2 |
| Fresh lemon | +9.9 |
| Tomato | +13.6 |
| Avocado  (protein) | +15.6 |

### Non-Stored Organic Grains and Legumes

| | |
|---|---|
| Buckwheat groats | +0.5 |
| Spelt | +0.5 |
| Lentils | +0.6 |
| Soy flour | +2.5 |

| | |
|---|---|
| Tofu | +3.2 |
| Lima beans | +12.0 |
| Soybeans, fresh | +12.0 |
| White beans (navy beans) | +12.1 |
| Granulated soy (cooked, ground soy beans) | +12.8 |
| Soy nuts (soaked soy beans, then air dried) | +26.5 |
| Soy lecithin, pure | +38.0 |

### Nuts

| | |
|---|---|
| Almonds | +3.6 |
| Brazil Nuts | -0.5 |

### Seeds

| | |
|---|---|
| Wheat kernel | -11.4 |
| Pumpkin seeds | -5.6 |
| Sunflower seeds | -5.4 |
| Flax seeds | -1.3 |
| Sesame seeds | +0.5 |
| Cumin seeds | +1.1 |
| Fennel seeds | +1.3 |
| Caraway seeds | +2.3 |

### Fats (Fresh, Cold-Pressed Oils)

| | |
|---|---|
| Olive oil | +1.0 |
| Borage oil | +3.2 |
| Flax seed oil | +3.5 |
| Evening primrose oil | +4.1 |
| Marine lipids | +4.7 |

### Water

| | |
|---|---|
| Distilled water | (neutral) |
| Coconut water | +9.04 |

# Foods You Can Eat Sparingly

**Fish**

| | |
|---|---|
| Fresh water fish | -11.8 |

**Fruits**

(In Season, for Cleansing only, or with Moderation)

| | |
|---|---|
| Rose hips | -15.5 |
| Pineapple | -12.6 |
| Mandarin orange | -11.5 |
| Banana, ripe | -10.1 |
| Pear | -9.9 |
| Peach | -9.7 |
| Apricot | -9.5 |
| Papaya | -9.4 |
| Orange | -9.2 |
| Mango | -8.7 |
| Tangerine | -8.5 |

| | |
|---|---|
| Currant | -8.2 |
| Gooseberry, ripe | -7.7 |
| Grape, ripe | -7.6 |
| Cranberry | -7.0 |
| Black currant | -6.1 |
| Strawberry | -5.4 |
| Blueberry | -5.3 |
| Raspberry | -5.1 |
| Yellow plum | -4.9 |
| Italian plum | -4.9 |
| Date | -4.7 |
| Cherry, sweet | -3.6 |
| Cantaloupe | -2.5 |
| Red currant | -2.4 |
| Fig juice powder | -2.4 |
| Grapefruit | -1.7 |
| Watermelon | -1.0 |

| | |
|---|---|
| Coconut, fresh | +0.5 |
| Cherry, sour | +3.5 |
| Banana, unripe | +4.8 |

**Non-Stored Grains**

| | |
|---|---|
| Brown rice | -12.5 |
| Wheat | -10.1 |

**Nuts**

| | |
|---|---|
| Walnuts | -8.0 |
| Macadamia Nuts | -3.2 |
| Hazelnuts | -2.0 |

**Fats**

| | |
|---|---|
| Sunflower oil | -6.7 |
| Coconut Milk | -1.5 |

# Foods You Should Never Eat

**Root Vegetables**

| | |
|---|---|
| Stored potatoes | +2.0 |

**Meat, Poultry and Fish**

| | |
|---|---|
| Pork | -38.0 |
| Veal | -35.0 |
| Beef | -34.5 |
| Ocean fish | -20.0 |
| Chicken | -18.0 |
| to -22.0 | |
| Eggs | -18.0 |
| to -22.0 | |
| Oysters | -5.0 |
| Liver | -3.0 |
| Organ meats | -3.0 |

**Milk and Milk Products**

| | |
|---|---|
| Hard cheese | -18.1 |
| Quark | -17.3 |
| Cream | -3.9 |
| Homogenized Milk | -1.0 |
| Buttermilk | +1.3 |

**Bread, Biscuits (Stored Grains/Risen Dough)**

| | |
|---|---|
| White bread | -10.0 |

| | |
|---|---|
| White biscuit | -6.5 |
| Whole-meal bread | -6.5 |
| Whole-grain bread | -4.5 |
| Rye bread | -2.5 |

**Nuts**

| | |
|---|---|
| Pistachios | -16.6 |
| Peanuts | -12.8 |
| Cashews | -9.3 |

**Fats**

| | |
|---|---|
| Margarine | -7.5 |
| Corn oil | -6.5 |
| Butter | -3.9 |

**Sweets**

| | |
|---|---|
| Artificial sweeteners | -26.5 |
| Chocolate | -24.6 |
| White sugar (refined cane sugar) | -17.6 |
| Beet sugar | -15.1 |
| Molasses | -14.6 |
| Dr. Bronner's Barley Malt Sweetener | -9.8 |
| Dried sugar cane juice (Sucanat) | -9.6 |
| Barley malt syrup | -9.3 |
| Fructose | -9.5 |
| Milk sugar | -9.4 |

| | |
|---|---|
| Turbinado sugar | -9.5 |
| Brown rice syrup | -8.7 |
| Honey | -7.6 |

**Condiments**

| | |
|---|---|
| Ketchup | -12.4 |
| Mayonnaise | -12.5 |
| Mustard | -19.2 |
| Soy sauce | -36.2 |
| Vinegar | -39.4 |

**Beverages**

| | |
|---|---|
| Liquor | -28.6 |
| to -38.7 | |
| Wine | -16.4 |
| Beer | -26.8 |
| Coffee | -25.1 |
| Fruit juice, packaged, natural | - 8.7 |
| Fruit juice sweetened with white sugar | -33.4 |
| Tea (black) | -27.1 |

**Miscellaneous**

Canned Foods
Processed Foods
Microwaved Food

# Table 2
## FUNGAL CONTENT OF CORN AND PEANUTS FOOD FROM FARMERS, MIDDLEMEN, AND RETAIL OULETS IN BANGKOK

*(Note: Surface was sterilized prior to fungal study.)*

Peanuts and corn are poisonous and carcinogens containing 25 mycotoxin-producing fungi. Researchers have reported the positive correlation of corn consumption and death from cancer of the esophagus and stomach. Peanuts have been associated with pancreatic and liver cancer. (Source: Young, Robert. *Sick and Tired?* Pleasant Grove, Utah: Woodland Publishing, 1999.)

**PEANUTS**

Aspergillus candidus
Aspergillus niger
Aspergillus wentii
Chaetomium funicola
Eurotium amstelodami
Eurotium repens
Fusarium equiseti
Fusarium solani
Macrophomina phaseolina
Penicillium aethiopicum
Penicillium funiculosum
Penicillium janthinellum
Penicillium pinophilum

Aspergillus flavus
Aspergillus tamarii
Chaetomium globosum
Chaetomium spp.
Eurotium chevalieri
Eurotium rubrum
Fusarium semitectum
Lasiodiplodia theobromae
Nigrospora oryzae
Penicillium citrinum
Penicillium glabrum
Penicillium olsonii
Rhizopus oryzae

**CORN**

Acremonium siricium
Aspergillus niger
Aspergillus wentii
Chaetomium globosum
Chaetomium spp.
Eurotium amstelodami
Eurotium rubrum
Fusarium proliferatum
Nigrospora oryzae
Penicillium pinophilum
Phoma spp.
Rhizopus oryzae
Trichoderma harzianum

Aspergillus flavus
Aspergillus tamarii
Bipolaris maydis
Chaetomium funicola
Curvularia lunata
Eurotium chevalieri
Fusarium moniliforme
Fusarium semitectum
Penicillium citrinum
Penicillium raistrickii
Rhizoctonia solani
Rhizopus arrhizus

# TABLE 3
## MICROFORM/SYMPTOGENIC LOAD COMPARISON OF FOODS

### Clean Plant Food:

Vegetables, fruits, legumes, seeds, nuts and sprouted grains (if uncontaminated in handling): 10 microorganisms/pathogens per gram.

### Animal Foods (for acceptable sale per U.S. Department of Agriculture):

Milk, Grade A Pasteurized: 20,000 microorganisms/pathogens per gram, or 5,000,000 per cup.

Butter: 300,000 to 1,000,000 microorganisms/ pathogens per gram, or 7,000,000 per patty.

Cheese: 300,000 to 1,000,000 microorganisms/ pathogens per gram, or 100,000,000 per serving.

Ice Cream: 300,000 to 1,000,000 microorganisms/pathogens per gram, or 225,000,000 per serving.

Eggs: 50,000 to 500,000 microorganisms/ pathogens per gram, or 37,500,000 per egg.

Beef, Poultry, Lamb, Pork, Seafood: 300,000 to 3,000,000 microorganisms/pathogens per gram, or 336,000,000 per serving.

Honey: 150,000 microorganisms/pathogens per gram.

*The average American meal of animal products contains 750,000,000–1,000,000,000 pleomorphic pathogenic microorganisms!*

*The average vegetarian meal consisting only of plant foods contains less than 500 pleomorphic pathogenic microorganisms.*

# Table 4
## CALCIUM, SODIUM, AND PROTEIN
## COMPOSITION OF ALKALIZING FOODS

*per 100 grams of edible portion*

| Food | Calcium | Sodium | Protein | Food | Calcium | Sodium | Protein |
|---|---|---|---|---|---|---|---|
| **Vegetables** | | | | Turnip Greens | 246 mg. | 49 mg. | 30% |
| Artichoke | 51 mg. | 43 mg. | 29% | Watercress | 151 mg. | 52 mg. | 22% |
| Asparagus | 23 mg. | 2 mg. | 25% | | | | |
| Bamboo Shoots | 13 mg. | 0 mg. | 26% | **Fruits** | | | |
| Beet Greens | 119 mg. | 130 mg. | 22% | Avocado (Calif.) | 10 mg. | 4 mg. | 22% |
| Broccoli | 103 mg. | 15 mg. | 49% | Avocado (Florida) | 10 mg. | 4 mg. | 13% |
| Brussels Sprouts | 36 mg. | 14 mg. | 49% | Cherry, Sour Red | 22 mg. | 2 mg. | 12% |
| Cabbage, Chinese | 43 mg. | 23 mg. | 12% | Cranberry | 14 mg. | 2 mg. | 4% |
| Cabbage, Red | 42 mg. | 26 mg. | 20% | Grapefruit, sour | 16 mg. | 1 mg. | 5% |
| Cauliflower | 25 mg. | 13 mg. | 27% | Lemon Juice | 7 mg. | 2 mg. | 5% |
| Celery | 39 mg. | 126 mg. | 10% | Tomato, red. | 13 mg. | 3 mg. | 11% |
| Chard, Swiss | 88 mg. | 147 mg. | 24% | Tomato, green | 13 mg. | 3 mg. | 12% |
| Chives | 69 mg. | 0 mg. | 18% | | | | |
| Collards (leaves) | 250 mg. | 0 mg. | 48% | **Legumes** | | | |
| Collards (stems) | 203 mg. | 43 mg. | 36% | Lima bean, fresh | 52 mg. | 2 mg. | 9% |
| Cress | 81 mg. | 14 mg. | 26% | Mung Sprouts | 118 mg. | 5 mg. | 38% |
| Cucumber | 25 mg. | 6 mg. | 10% | Red bean, dried | 110 mg. | 10 mg. | 23% |
| Dandelion greens | 187 mg. | 76 mg. | 27% | Chickpea | 150 mg. | 26 mg. | 21% |
| Eggplant | 12 mg. | 2 mg. | 12% | Lentil, dried | 79 mg. | 30 mg. | 25% |
| Fennel | 100 mg. | 0 mg. | 28% | Pea, green fresh | 26 mg. | 2 mg. | 6% |
| Garlic | 29 mg. | 19 mg. | 62% | Soybean, fresh | 67 mg. | 0 mg. | 11% |
| Kale (leaves) | 249 mg. | 75 mg. | 60% | Soybean, dried | 226 mg. | 5 mg. | 34% |
| Kale (stem) | 179 mg. | 75 mg. | 42% | Soybean Sprouts | 48 mg. | 0 mg. | 6% |
| Leek | 52 mg. | 5 mg | 22% | | | | |
| Lettuce, Boston | 35 mg. | 9 mg. | 12% | **Nuts and Seeds** | | | |
| Lettuce, Loose-leaf | 68 mg. | 9 mg. | 13% | Almond | 234 mg. | 4 mg. | 19% |
| Lettuce, Iceberg | 20 mg. | 9 mg. | 27% | Brazil Nut | 186 mg. | 1 mg. | 14% |
| Mustard Greens | 183 mg. | 32 mg. | 22% | Filbert | 209 mg. | 2 mg. | 13% |
| Okra | 92 mg. | 0 mg. | 24% | Pumpkin Seed | 51 mg. | 0 mg. | 29% |
| Onion (Green) | 51 mg. | 5 mg. | 15% | Sesame Seed | 1160 mg. | 60 mg. | 19% |
| Parsley | 203 mg. | 45 mg. | 36% | Sunflower Seed | 120 mg. | 30 mg. | 24% |
| Pepper, Red | 13 mg. | 0 mg. | 14% | | | | |
| Pepper, Green | 9 mg. | 13 mg. | 12% | **Grains** | | | |
| Pepper, Red Hot | 130 mg. | 373 mg. | 13% | Barley | 34 mg. | 0 mg. | 10% |
| Radish | 30 mg. | 18 mg. | 10% | Millet | 20 mg. | 5 mg. | 10% |
| Rhubarb | 96 mg. | 2 mg. | 11% | Rice, Brown | 32 mg. | 9 mg. | 8% |
| Seaweed, Dulse | 296 mg. | 2085 mg. | 25% | Wheat | 46 mg. | 3 mg. | 14% |
| Seaweed, Agar | 567 mg. | 0 mg. | 0% | Wheat Bran | 119 mg. | 9 mg. | 16% |
| Spinach | 93 mg. | 71 mg. | 45% | | | | |

# Table 5
## SPROUTING GUIDE

| Seed | Quantity | Soak time (hrs) | Rinse/Drain (# daily) | Time to harvest | Days/In. | Suggested Uses |
|---|---|---|---|---|---|---|
| Alfalfa | (2 Tbs.) | 6 to 8 | 2 | 3 to 6 days | 1 to 2" | Salads, sandwiches, juices |
| Chinese Cabbage | (1 cup) | 6 to 8 | 2 | 3 to 4 days | 1/2 to 1" | Salads and juices |
| Fenugreek | (1 cup) | 6 to 8 | 2 to 3 | 3 to 4 days | 1/2 to 1" | Salads and snacks |
| Garbanzo | (1 cup) | 16 | 2 to 3 | 3 to 6 days | 1/8 to 1" | Salads, soups, casseroles |
| Lentil | (1 cup) | 8 to 12 | 2 to 3 | 2 to 4 days | 1/2 to 1" | Salads, soups, steam-fry |
| Mung Bean | (1/2 cup) | 8 to 12 | 2 to 3 | 2 to 4 days | 1/2 to 1" | Salads, soups, steam-fry |
| Peas | (1/2 or 1 cup) | 8 to 12 | 2 to 3 | 2 to 3 days | 1/2 to 1" | Salads, soups, steam-fry |
| Radish | (2 Tbs. or 1 cup) | 6 to 8 | 2 | 3 to 4 days | 1/2 to 1" | Salads, juices, sandwiches |
| Red Clover | (2 Tbs.) | 8 | 2 | 3 to 6 days | 1/2 to 2" | Salads, juices, sandwiches |
| Sesame | (1/4 cup) | 8 | 2 | 1 to 3 days | 0 to 1" | Breads, snacks, casseroles |
| Soybean | (1/2 or 1 cup) | 16 | 3 | 3 to 5 days | 1/2 to 1" | Casseroles, soups, steam-fry |
| Sunflower, hulled | (1/2 or 1 cup) | 6 to 8 | 2 | 1 to 2 days | 0 to 1/2" | Salads and snacks |

# Table 6
## RECIPE SUBSTITUTIONS

***If a Recipe Calls For . . . Substitute With:***

A. 1 pkg. of yeast . . . 1 tsp. of non-aluminum baking powder

B. Whole wheat or white flour . . . Try spelt, buckwheat, millet flour, or combinations

C. Milk . . . Soy milk, Rice Dream®, almond milk, sesame milk

D. Vinegar . . . Equal amounts of lemon or lime juice

E. Soy sauce or tamari . . . Bragg™ Liquid Aminos

F. Regular cooking oils or salad oil . . . Good oils such as olive, sunflower, flax seed, borage, almond, grape seed, or Udo's Choice®

G. Cheese . . . Sprouts

H. Meat . . . Tofu products (without yeast)

I. Eggs . . . Egg Replacer (as directed on package)

J. Salt . . . Real Salt™ or Celtic Sea Salt™

K. Walnuts or cashew nuts . . . Almonds, hazelnuts, pecans, pine nuts

L. Butter or margarine . . . Good oils like olive oil, flax seed oil, or Udo's Choice®

M. White rice . . . Organic brown rice, brown or natural white basmati rice, spelt, buckwheat groats, millet, kamut, quinoa, amaranth

N. Bread . . . Unleavened, yeast-free, sprouted breads

O. Regular wheat pasta . . . Vegetable, spelt, or artichoke pasta

# Glossary of Terms

**Acid:** A compound capable of donating a hydrogen ion (proton) to a base. A product of fermentation by microforms, degenerative to body substances, cells and tissues.

**Aduki bean:** A legume, also called "adzuki bean." The small seeds of a bushy annual plant native to China, aduki beans are a popular ingredient in Chinese and Japanese cooking.

**Agar:** Gelling and thickening agent of plant origin, made from the cell wall of red algae.

**Alkaline:** Relating to, containing, or having the reaction of an alkali base.

**Almonds:** Particularly rich in protein, iron, calcium, vitamin B2 and vitamin E. Almonds make a very good milk, and butter when ground. Soaking hydrates them for a wonderful crunchy snack.

**Ash residue:** The by-product of food and energy metabolism, which can be neutral, acid, or alkaline.

**Amino acids:** The constituents of proteins, eight of which are essential to the human body. Without them, severe metabolic and growth disorders result.

**Black beans:** Kidney shaped with a shiny skin and white center, these beans are grown widely in South America. Sometimes called "turtle beans."

**Brazil nuts:** Rich in protein, the B vitamin thiamine, and magnesium. Brazil nuts have a creamy texture and a delicate flavor that makes them excellent for eating raw in salads or snacks.

**Buckwheat:** Not a cereal but rather a simple variety of bistort with triangular seeds whose contents are nonetheless like those of a cereal. Contains protein and many minerals as well as lysine, an essential amino acid that rarely occurs in cereals. Buckwheat is desirable because it contains no gluten and is considered low fungal.

**Chlorophyll:** The green coloring in plants, chlorophyll plays an essential role in photosynthesis and is thought to be a genuine elixir of health.

**Cranberry beans:** Also known as "Shelly beans" in Indiana and Ohio. This bean has a much sweeter and more delicate flavor than the pinto bean. When cooked it loses its markings and becomes solid in color. Great in soups, side dishes, and pasta dishes.

**Flax seeds:** Flax seeds are very high in omega-3 and omega-6 essential fats. They are available in most health-food stores. They can be ground or soaked, and are used also as a thickener.

**Food combining:** Nutritional fundamental rules for combining compatible foods together for optimum health.

**Garbanzo beans:** An annual bush with short pods; its beans are light beige-yellow. Used in Africa, Spain and India to make flour, hummus, purees, stews and vegetable accompaniments. Also known as chickpeas.

**Hazelnuts:** A good source of vitamin E and low in fat, also known as "filberts." Hazelnuts can also be soaked like almonds.

**Kamut:** An older cereal variety from Ancient Egypt with grains often three times the size of wheat. High protein content as well as being rich in amino acids and vitamins. Provides a robust nutty flavor.

**Kidney beans:** Red color and kidney shape make these beans distinctive, as does their fine aroma. Very popular in South America. Very high in fiber and good for soups and salads.

**Kuzu Root:** Also known as "kudzu." A natural jelling and thickening agent made from a root that grows wild in Japan.

**Lentils:** Small legumes, rich in protein, iron, calcium, and B vitamins. Can be used for sprouting. Available in many colors, green and red being the most common.

**Macadamia nuts:** These nuts are expensive and very creamy. They are usually sold roasted and salted. Try to buy them raw and freeze them for a longer shelf life.

**Microzyma:** An organized ferment. An independently living, imperishable fundamental anatomical element. Capable of multiplying, it is the basic form from which organisms are constituted, and to which they are reduced upon death.

**Microforms:** A general term for microscopic life forms. It covers everything from microzymas to mold, beneficial to harmful.

**Millet:** The oldest cultivated variety of cereal in the world and an important basic foodstuff in Africa and Central Asia, as well as being used widely in Europe. Very rich in unsaturated fatty acids and vitamins and good as a rice substitute.

**Monounsaturated fats:** Generally found in oil, they are present in practically all foods that contain fat, both animal and vegetable. They are generally liquid at room temperature and can be metabolized by the body. They are used mainly as good energy-burning fat in the body.

**Mung beans:** Cultivated in China and India, where they are known as "mungdal." They are also made into bean sprouts.

**Nori:** Popular green seaweed that comes in square sheet, used for making sushi.

**Olive oil:** This oil is mostly associated with Mediterranean cuisine, and is easily digested and has a positive effect on the stomach and intestines. It is also known to reduce the risk of heart and circulatory diseases. It has a broad range of flavors, depending on the type of olive, time of harvest, the climate, and type of soil. It should not be refrigerated but should be stored in a cool, dark place. It keeps very well for nine to twelve months.

**Pecans:** Pecans offer a delicious mealy texture which is good in salads, wraps, and warmed nut loafs. They can also be soaked with good results.

**pH:** The symbol expressing the degree of alkalinity or acidity of a solution. A solution with pH of 7 is neutral; values below 7 indicate a degree of acidity; values above 7 indicate a degree of alkalinity. The normal pH of blood serum is approximately 7.3 and the normal pH of the urine is 6.8.

**Pinenuts:** Protein-rich pinenuts, also known as "pignoli" or "piñons," are soft, white, creamy-colored nuts taken from the pine cone of the piñon tree. Store in the freezer, as these nuts have a very short shelf-life.

**Pleomorphism:** The principle that microforms are not fixed species, as are higher animals and plants, but can rapidly change both form and function during a life cycle. The occurrence of various shapes in the same developmental phase or form.

**Polyunsaturated fats:** Like linoleic acid (bi-saturated), linolenic acid (tri-saturated) and arachidon acid (vitamin F). Usually vegetable fats, they are liquid, react easily and are essential for human organisms. They help the body regulate all its functions, and as the body cannot produce these fats, they are an important part of the diet.

**Pumpkin seeds:** Sometimes called "pita seeds," pumpkin seeds are particularly rich in minerals, especially zinc. They are a good addition to any meal. Soaking plumps them and softens their taste.

**Quinoa:** A plant that grows in the Andes at altitudes in excess of 13,000 feet (4000 meters). Nutritious as a leaf vegetable and having small seeds rich in vitamins and other nutrients, it was much prized by the Incas. When used as flour, it can be bitter because it contains saporin. Mostly available in health food stores.

**Rice:** Asia's main foodstuff that loses its nutrients when milled and polished to produce white rice. However, Basmati rice is a naturally occurring white rice. Hulled, natural brown rice or whole-grain rice contain all eight essential amino acids, vitamins and minerals. Because of extensive use of pesticides, it is advisable only to use organic, whole-grain rice.

**Saturated fats:** These include palmitin, stearin and butyric acid. They are found in all animal fats and also in palm and coconut oil; additionally, they are produced in the human body. They are often solid at room temperature, do not react and are very hard to digest.

**Sesame seeds:** Rich in B3, iron, protein and zinc, sesame seeds are usually white but may be brown, red or black, depending on the variety. Tahini is a butter made from ground sesame seeds.

**Spelt:** This form of wheat has highly nutritious gluten and is recommended as a good alternative grain, since virtually all spelt is grown organically.

**Sunflower seeds:** Nutritionally speaking, sunflower seeds are a good source of vitamins B1, B6, and potassium. They also produce a hearty sprout that is high in protein.

**Tofu:** Soybean product obtained by coagulation.

**UDO's:** The brand name for an oil blend developed by Udo Erasmus, author of *Fats that Heal, Fats that Kill*. A blend of unrefined oils consisting of flax, sunflower, sesame and evening primrose. Found in the refrigerated sections of most health food stores.

# Shelley Young's
## ACADEMY OF CULINARY ARTS
*Where the Science of Food meets the Taste of Health!*

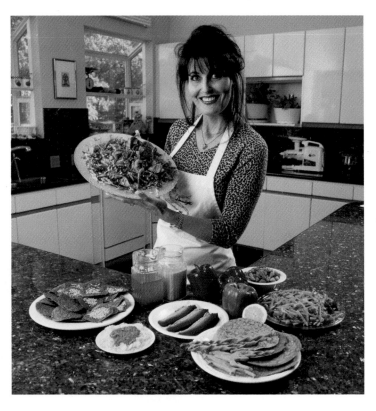

***Come and learn*** how to prepar
beautiful alkalizing meals wit
Shelley Redford Young. Thes
informative, instructional work
shops are held 4 times a year i
Shelley's beautiful mountain hom
in Alpine, Utah.

***Join her to learn*** how easy and fas
alkalizing meals can be prepared
Salads, soups, healthy snacks an
delicious vegan entrees, with
nutritious alkalizing meal served a
the end of class. Call now t
reserve your spot in a class, as siz
is limited.

*It's all education and entertainment at Shelley Young's cooking workshops!*

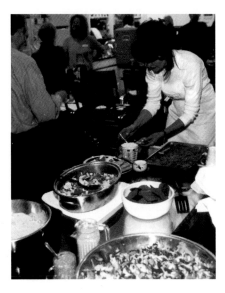
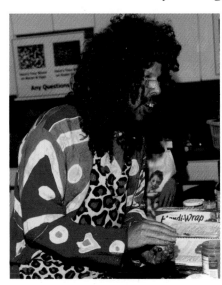
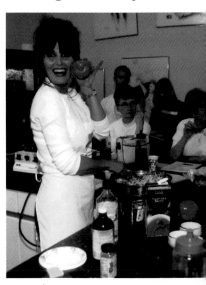

## *To enroll now in Shelley's Classes, call*
# 800-876-5403 or 801-756-7850